Get Through
MRCGP: New MCQ Module

Una Coales

MD FRCS FRCSOto DRCOG DFFP MRCGP
GP Registrar, London Deanery, Department of Postgraduate
General Practice Education, London, UK

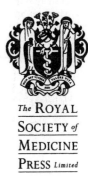

The ROYAL
SOCIETY of
MEDICINE
PRESS Limited

Royal Society of Medicine Press Ltd

Published by the Royal Society of Medicine Press Ltd
1 Wimpole Street, London W1G 0AE, UK
Tel: +44 (0)20 7290 2921
Fax: +44 (0)20 7290 2929
E-mail: publishing@rsm.ac.uk
Website: www.rsmpress.co.uk

British Library Cataloguing in Publication Data
A catalogue record for this book is available from the British Library

ISBN 1-85315-570-5

Distribution in Europe and Rest of World:
Marston Book Services Ltd
PO Box 269
Abingdon
Oxon OX14 4YN, UK
Tel: +44 (0)1235 465500
Fax: +44 (0)1235 465555

Distribution in the USA and Canada:
Royal Society of Medicine Press Ltd
c/o Jamco Distribution Inc
1401 Lakeway Drive
Lewisville, TX 75057, USA
Tel: +1 800 538 1287
Fax: +1 972 353 1303
E-mail: jamco@majors.com

Distribution in Australia and New Zealand:
MacLennan + Petty Pty Ltd
Suite 405, 152 Bunnerong Road
Eastgardens NSW 2036, Australia
Tel: + 61 2 9349 5811
Fax: + 61 2 9349 5911

Phototypeset by Phoenix Photosetting, Chatham, Kent
Printed in Great Britain by Bell and Bain Ltd, Glasgow

Contents

Preface

In the Spring of 2002, the Royal College of General Practitioners introduced the first of the new MCQ modules of the MRCGP exam. No longer are the questions in true/false format, but now include single best answers, multiple best answers, sentence completions, algorithms and extended matching questions. There is no negative marking, so GUESS!

I have sat and passed this new module, and by consulting colleagues who have also sat it, by reading all the hot topics in the weekly *BMJ* and *GP* magazines, by consulting current NICE/NSF guidelines and by reviewing royal college guidelines into the management of chronic disease, I have managed to produce three sample exam papers for you to practise and revise for this new module. This will be the only revision book you will need!

As a bonus, I have also included a chapter of tips for the MRCGP written paper module, which I was also fortunate to pass at my first sitting as a GP SHO. The good news is that by passing the MRCGP MCQ module, you will get credit for the COGPED MCQ paper required for summative assessment in your registrar year. For those who are not keen on completing audit cycles, I have included a copy of the discussion paper I submitted to pass the NPMS marking schedule, which can be taken in lieu of an audit. And finally, I suggest you make use of the single MRCGP/SA video route to complete the three requirements for summative assessment in your busy registrar year. Then you can relax in month 11, as your GP trainer completes the trainer's report.

Una Coales
GP Registrar, London Deanery

Recommended texts and references

American Psychiatric Association (2000). *Diagnostic and Statistic Manual of Mental Disorders, Text Revision (DSM-IV-TR)*, 4th edn. American Psychiatric Association, Washington, DC.

BMA/RPS (2003). *British National Formulary*. British Medical Associaton/Royal Pharmaceutical Society of Great Britain, London.

British Medical Journals (2002–2003). BMJ Publishing Group, London.

Collier J, Longmore M, Scally P (2003). *Oxford Handbook of Clinical Specialties*, 6th edn. Oxford University Press, Oxford.

Davies T, Craig TKJ (1998). *ABC of Mental Health*. BMJ Publishing Group, London.

Department of Health (1999). *Drug Misuse and Dependence – Guidelines on Clinical Management*. HMSO, London.

Fitzpatrick TB, Johnson RA, Wolff K, Suurmond R (2000). *Color Atlas and Synopsis of Clinical Dermatology*, 4th edn. McGraw-Hill, New York.

Glasier A, Gebbie A, Loudon N (2000). *Handbook of Family Planning and Reproductive Healthcare*, 4th edn. Churchill Livingstone, London.

Harrington JM, Gill FS, Aw TC, Gardiner K (1998). *Pocket Consultant: Occupational Health,* 4th edn. Blackwell Publishing, Oxford.

Jenkins R *et al.* (2000). *WHO Guide to Mental Health in Primary Care.* The Royal Society of Medicine Press, London.

Kilburn J (2000). *Answer Plans for the MRCGP*. BIOS Scientific Publishers, Oxford.

Kumar PJ, Clark ML (2002). *Clinical Medicine*, 5th edn. Baillière Tindall, London.

Lattimer CR, Wilson NM, Lagatolla NRF (2002). *Key Topics in General Surgery*, 2nd edn. BIOS Scientific Publishers, Oxford.

Longmore JM, Wilkinson I, Torok E (2001). *Oxford Handbook of Clinical Medicine*, 5th edn. Oxford University Press, Oxford.

McLatchie GR, Leaper D (2001). *Oxford Handbook of Clinical Surgery*, 2nd edn. Oxford University Press, Oxford.

Roland NJ, McRae RDR, McMombe AW (2000). *Key Topics in Otolaryngology*, 2nd edn. BIOS Scientific Publishers, Oxford.

Solomon L, Nayagam D, Warwick D (2001). *Apley's System of Orthopaedics and Fractures*, 8th edn. Arnold, London.

1. For which of the following conditions does the Department of Health recommend pneumococcal vaccination?

   A diabetes mellitus
   B nephrotic syndrome
   C coeliac syndrome
   D asplenia
   E cirrhosis

2. Viagra is licensed on the NHS and endorsed as 'SLS' to treat erectile dysfunction in men who have?

   A Parkinson's disease
   B renal transplant
   C prostate cancer
   D diabetes mellitus
   E multiple sclerosis

3–7. Anatomy of the tympanic membrane

   A pars tensa
   B pars flaccida
   C stapedius
   D incus
   E manubrium of malleus
   F uncus
   G light reflex

   Label the parts of the tympanic membrane shown below from the list above:

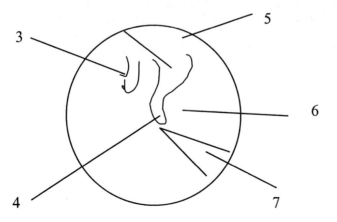

8–14. Match the following child development milestones:

A 6 weeks
B 12 weeks
C 6 months
D 7 months
E 8 months
F 9 months
G 12 months
H 18 months
I 2 years
J 3 years
K 4 years
L 5 years

8. Able to transfer cube from hand to hand.

9. Able to sit without support.

10. Able to hop on one foot.

11. Follows object 1 metre away.

12. Able to speak 10–12 words.

13. Knows first and last name.

14. Turns head to sounds level with the ear.

15–19. Fitness to drive

A no driving licence restrictions
B I month off driving
C 6 months off driving
D 12 months off driving
F permanently barred and requires DVLA notification
G refusal or revocation
H driving must cease until cause identified
I relicensing when symptom-free for 6/52

Match the following scenarios with the appropriate fitness-to-drive regulations:

15. A 32-year-old bus driver is diagnosed as HIV-positive.

16. A 40-year-old HGV driver presents with chest pain. He is referred for an exercise stress test and is able to complete 3 stages of the Bruce protocol on exercise–stress test without anti-anginal medication and is free from signs of cardiovascular dysfunction.

17. A 40-year-old IVDA reports that he blacked out at the wheel and hit a tree. He has had no further episodes of syncope. He states that his tongue is sore.

18. A 55-year-old man has suffered a myocardial infarction. He has been treated and has undergone CABG.

19. A 50-year-old woman suffers a single episode of TIA and weakness in her left arm. She recovers.

20. Initial treatment recommendation for scabies is as follows:
    A Apply malathion 0.5% preparation over entire body after a hot bath and wash off after 12 hours. Repeat in 1 week's time.
    B Apply benzoyl benzoate over the whole body, repeat without bathing on the following day and wash off 24 hours later. Repeat for up to 3 consecutive days.
    C Apply permethrin 5% dermal cream over whole body and wash off after 12 hours. Repeat in 1 week's time.
    D Prescribe ivermectin as a single dose of 200 μg/kg by mouth.
    E Apply carbaryl lotion over whole body after hot bath and wash off after 24 hours. Repeat once a week for 3 consecutive weeks.

21–25. Sickness certificates

    A med 3
    B med 4
    C med 5
    D med 6
    E RM7
    F DS 1500

21. This statement is completed if the doctor doubts the incapacity of the patient.

22. This statement of incapacity to work allows a return-to-work date to be given not more than 2 weeks after the date of the examination.

23. This statement is requested prior to a Personal Capacity Assessment.

24. This statement is for backdated medical certificates on the basis of a recent written report from another doctor.

25. This statement is issued for patients with terminal illness, who are likely to die within 6 months.

26–32. Match the following Sections of the Mental Health Act:

A Section 2
B Section 3
C Section 4
D Section 5
E Section 7
F Section 115
G Section 135
H Section 136

26. This gives police the right to remove a person from a public place to a place of safety, ie a prison cell or hospital, for 72 hours to permit medical examination.

27. This gives a social worker the right of entry into a person's premises.

28. This allows one doctor to detain an inpatient for up to 72 hours in an emergency situation. A psychiatrist must then be contacted.

29. This permits compulsory emergency admission to hospital for 72 hours and requires one doctor who has seen the person in the last 24 hours plus a social worker or family member.

30. This requires 2 doctors (one of whom is section 12-approved) to admit a patient to hospital for up to 28 days for assessment and is not renewable.

31. This gives police the right of entry into premises to remove a person to a place of safety under a magistrate's warrant.

32. This requires 2 doctors (one of whom is section 12-approved) to admit a patient to hospital for up to 6 months for treatment and is renewable.

33–39. Algorithm for Dyspepsia according to the British Society of Gastroenterology

A 45 years
B 50 years
C 55 years
D endoscopy
E double-contrast barium meal (DCBM)
F *H. pylori* serology
G urea breath test
H triple therapy for *H. pylori*
I antacids
J PPI

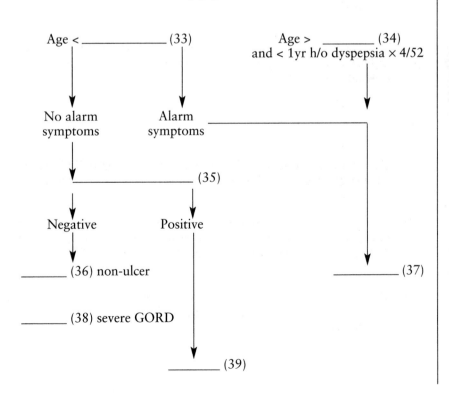

Dyspepsia

40. According to the British Thoracic Society Guidelines for the Management of Stable COPD, the following treatment is advised for a 45-year-old man with breathlessness on exertion, cough and a 39% predicted FEV1.

A regular combined inhaled short-acting β_2-agonists and anticholinergics and 30 mg oral prednisolone for 2 weeks

B regular inhaled short-acting β_2-agonists or regular inhaled anticholinergics and consider corticosteroid therapy

C theophylline and long-term oxygen therapy

D regular combined inhaled short-acting β_2-agonists and anticholinergics, corticosteroid trial and antibiotic therapy

E regular inhaled short-acting β_2-agonists and regular inhaled anticholinergics, corticosteroid therapy and long-acting β_2-agonists

41. Specialist referral in the management of COPD is required in the following situations:

A bullous lung disease

B cor pulmonale

C uncertain diagnosis

D family history of α_1-antitrypsin deficiency

E oxygen therapy

42. Which evidence-based questionnaire is recommended for postnatal depression?

A Beck

B Edinburgh

C Hamilton

D Glasgow

E CAGE

43. Guidelines for urgent urology referral include:

A swellings in the body of the testis

B palpable renal masses

C an elevated age-specific PSA in men with a 10-year life expectancy without signs of an active UTI

D painful macroscopic haematuria in adults

E microscopic haematuria in adults over 50 years with irritative voiding symptoms

44. Guidelines for urgent referral to colorectal clinic include:

A rectal bleeding and change in bowel habits in patients over 50 years of age

B rectal bleeding and/or change in bowel habits in patients over 40 with ulcerative colitis

C iron deficiency anaemia with a normal upper endoscopy and a Hb of < 10 g/dl

D change in bowel habits in a patient over 40 with previous polyps

E an easily palpable renal mass

45. Cervical pap smear is recommended every 3 years for women between the ages of:

A 18–60
B 20–62
C 20–64
D 20–65
E 22–70

46. Breast cancer screening with mammography is recommended for women between the ages of:

A 40–60
B 45–60
C 45–65
D 50–60
E 50–64

47–51. Match the following ENT conditions:

A acoustic neuroma
B occupational noise damage
C presbyacusis
D otosclerosis
E Ménière's disease
F herpes zoster oticus

47. A 35-year-old pregnant woman presents with bilateral conductive hearing loss. Her TMs appear normal.

48. A 70-year-old man presents with gradual onset of bilateral sensorineural hearing loss.

49. A 65-year-old woman presents with sudden onset of unilateral facial weakness and sensorineural hearing loss. She is also noted to have vesicles in the external auditory meatus.

50. A 50-year-old woman presents with unilateral low-frequency sensorineural hearing loss and vertigo.

51. A 50-year-old man presents with gradual onset of unilateral sensorineural hearing loss and unilateral tinnitus.

52–56. Match the following drugs with the list of side-effects:

A orange-red tears
B dry eyes
C double vision
D altered colour vision
E cataract

52. Sildenafil.

53. Propranolol.

54. Carbamazepine.

55. Prednisolone.

56. Rifampicin.

57–62. Match the following consultation models:

A Byrne and Long
B John Heron
C Roger Neighbour
D D. Pendleton
E M. Balint
F Eric Berne
G Stott and Davis

57. Connecting, summarizing, handing over, safety netting and housekeeping.

58. Management of present problems, modification of help-seeking behaviours, management of continuing problems and opportunistic health promotion.

59. Define the reason for the patient's attendance, consider other problems, choose an appropriate action with the patient, achieve a shared understanding, involve the patient in the management plan, use time and resources appropriately and establish a relationship with the patient that helps to achieve other tasks.

60. A study of 2500 audiotaped consultations identifying 'doctor-centred' and 'patient-centred' behaviours.

61. The spontaneous or dependent child, the logical adult, and the critical or caring parent.

62. The doctor as a drug, the child as the presenting complaint, elimination by appropriate physical examination, collusion of anonymity, the flash and the mutual investment company.

63. The Royal College of Physicians Guidelines for Oxygen Therapy recommend use of long-term oxygen therapy after specialist assessment for the following conditions:

    A obstructive sleep apnoea despite continuous positive airways pressure therapy
    B pulmonary hypertension without parenchymal lung involvement when $PaO_2 < 8$ kPa
    C cystic fibrosis when $PaO_2 < 7.3$ kPa
    D COPD with $PaO_2 < 7.3$ kPa (on air)
    E pulmonary malignancy with dyspnoea on moderate exertion

64. Contraindications to aromatherapy include which of the following (multiple best answer)?

    A first-trimester pregnancy
    B epilepsy
    C hypertension
    D homeopathy
    E exposure to the sun
    F contact dermatitis

65. Which of the following statements regarding immunization are correct?

A Anaphylactic reaction to egg ingestion contraindicates influenza and yellow fever vaccines.

B Anaphylactic reaction to egg ingestion contraindicates MMR vaccine.

C A personal or family history of inflammatory bowel disease contraindicates MMR vaccine.

D Children given recent oral poliomyelitis vaccine should not be taken swimming.

E Children given recent oral poliomyelitis vaccine contraindicates tonsillectomy.

66. Which of the following statement(s) regarding homeopathy is/are correct?

A Homeopathy was developed into a system of medicine by Dr Samuel Hahnemann in the late 18th century.

B Belladonna is suggested for toothaches.

C There are no contraindications to the use of homeopathy.

D The principle of homeopathy uses the Law of Similars; ie when a substance used in large doses causes symptoms, in minute doses, it can cure.

E Homeopathy offers an alternative to the MMR vaccine.

67–72. Match the following distribution graphs:

A positively skewed
B negatively skewed
C normal
D equal mean but different variances
E equal variances but different means
F bimodal

67.

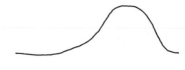

68.

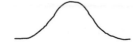

69.

70.

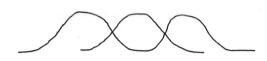

71.

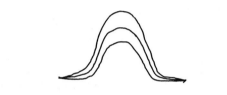

72.

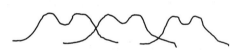

73–78. Hormone replacement therapy

    A oestradiol patches 50 µg
    B oestradiol pessary
    C combined oestrogen/progesterone
    D tibolone
    E continuous combined HRT
    F raloxifene

For each of the patients below, select from the list of options above the **single** most appropriate treatment option.

73. A 50-year-old woman requests 'no period' HRT. She is 1 year post-menopausal and also reports low libido and low mood.

74. A 60-year-old woman complains of atrophic vaginitis.

75. A 55-year-old woman requests HRT for hot flushes. She has had a hysterectomy.

76. A 50-year-old woman requests HRT but she does not want to see the return of her periods. She is 1 year postmenopausal.

77. A 60-year-old woman noted to have a kyphotic spine requests HRT.

78. A 40-year-old woman is confirmed to have premature menopause with elevated serum LH and FSH levels.

79–82. Dermatological conditions

A leukoplakia
B scabies
C body lice
D lichen sclerosus
E lichen planus
F contact dermatitis
G eczema
H psoriasis

For each of the patients below, select from the list of options above the **single** most likely diagnosis.

79. A 40-year-old hairdresser presents with an itchy rash on her inner wrists. The lesions are small reddish-purple papules and appear in linear form.

80. An 80-year-old female resident of a nursing home presents with an itchy generalized rash over her body, which spares her face. She reports that the itching is worse at night. On examination, she has an itchy papular rash with isolated vesicles on her hands.

81. A 50-year-old heavy smoker presents with a white lesion on the undersurface of his tongue.

82. A 28-year-old female who smokes 20 cigs/day presents with linear plaques and palmar pustulosis.

83–87. Match the following clinical scenarios with the appropriate timing of introduction of contraception after giving birth:

A immediately
B day 21
C 4 weeks
D 6 weeks
E 8 weeks
F delayed until after baby's first birthday

83. A 35-year-old female decides she would like the progestogen-only pill form of contraception. She intends to breastfeed. She has no contraindications to the POP.

84. A 25-year-old female would like the Depo-Provera injection. She intends to breastfeed and has no contraindications to injectables.

85. A 44-year-old female would like sterilization after the birth of her 6th child.

86. A 40-year-old female would like the Mirena IUS fitted after the birth of her 3rd child.

87. A 30-year-old female would like to start Microgynon after giving birth. She intends to bottle-feed and has no contraindications to the COC.

88–96. National Service Framework for Coronary Heart Disease issued by the Department of Health

Fill in the spaces using the words from the list below:

A I
B V
C north
D south
E African
F Indian
G low-dose aspirin
H blood pressure
I <130/80
J <140/85
K statins
L ACE inhibitors
M warfarin or aspirin
N beta-blockers
O HbAIC
P spironolactone

CHD is the single commonest cause of premature death in the UK. Men of working age in social class _____ (88) are 50% more likely to die from CHD than men in the population as a whole. Death rates are higher for people living in the _____ (89) of the country. For people born in the _____ (90) subcontinent, the death rate from heart disease is 38% higher for men and 43% higher for women than rates for the country as a whole. People with diagnosed CHD or other occlusive arterial disease should be offered daily _____ (91) medication and advice and treatment to maintain a BP _____ (92). People who also have left ventricular dysfunction should be offered _____ (93). People who have also had an MI should be started on _____ (94). People over 60 years old who also have atrial fibrillation should commence _____ (95). Meticulous control of _____ (96) is advised for people who also have diabetes.

97–101. Match the following heart failure trials with their respective descriptions:

A ELITE
B CIBIS II
C RALES
D SOLVD
E CONSENSUS
F MERIT-HF

97. This study published in the *NEJM* in 1999 looked at a large RCT of people with NYHA class III/IV grade of heart failure on treatment including an ACE inhibitor, and found that adding an aldosterone receptor antagonist (spironolactone) further decreased mortality.

98. This study published in the *Lancet* in 1997 found that losartan in the elderly reduces symptoms of heart failure and mortality.

99. This trial published in the *Lancet* in 1999 found that long-term use of a beta-blocker, ie bisoprolol, in combination with ACE inhibitors in patients with NYHA class III/IV grade of heart failure reduced mortality.

100. This trial published in the *NEJM* in 2001 showed that adding enalapril to people on conventional treatment with NYHA class II/III heart failure improves symptoms, reduces mortality and reduces hospital admissions.

101. Published in the *Lancet* in 1999, this trial is the largest randomized, double-blind, placebo-controlled, multicentred study of β_1-blockade in heart failure, with 3991 patients treated. The study was conducted in 13 countries in Europe and the USA. This study showed that long-term use of metoprolol CR/XL, in addition to standard therapy including an ACE inhibitor, reduced total mortality and hospitalization by 31% in people with symptoms compatible with NYHA class II/III.

102–110. GP Fees and Allowances & Superannuation

Match the following services with the appropriate payment category:

A items of service payments
B reimbursement
C practice allowances
D private medical work
E capitation fees

102. Contraceptive service fee.

103. Maternity medical services (MMS).

104. Rural practice payments.

105. Dispensing payments.

106. Initial practice allowance.

107. Childhood immunizations.

108. Night visit payments.

109. Cremation fees.

110. Child health surveillance fee.

111–115. Squint

Match the following definitions with the correct type of squint:

A latent squint
B pseudosquint
C esotropia
D exotropia
E paralytic

111. This is the commonest type in children and may be due to hypermetropia. Amblyopia may be a problem. One eye is turned in (convergent).

112. This is often intermittent and tends to occur in older children. Amblyopia is unlikely. One eye is turned out.

113. Diplopia is most marked when trying to look in the direction of the pull of the affected muscle.

114. Prominent epicanthal folds with a central and symmetrical corneal reflection from a bright light.

115. This squint is demonstrated by movement of the covered eye as the cover is removed during the cover test.

116–124. Types of study designs

Fill in the spaces using the appropriate word from the list below:

A cross-sectional
B case–control
C cohort
D randomized controlled
E null hypothesis
F p-value
G odds ratio
H confidence interval
I confounding factor
J relative risk
K incidence

A _____ (116) study is a retrospective study that looks for exposure or presence of a factor association and not causation. It cannot calculate the incidence of a disease but can calculate the _____ (117) under certain conditions.

A _____ (118) study is a prospective study and can calculate incidence of disease directly, relative and attributable risk.

A _____ (119) study is descriptive in nature and provides a snapshot of the population in question. It cannot assess _____ (120).

A _____ (121) study gives the best evidence of cause and effect. It is an intervention study based on findings of observational studies.

A positive _____ (122) makes an association more extreme and leads to misleading association between two factors.

A narrow _____ (123) indicates less chance of sample variability and suggests greater certainty.

A _____ (124) of 1 indicates that there is no association between the exposure and the outcome.

125. Which of the following occupational chemical exposures are correctly linked with their respective diseases?

A vinyl chloride and hepatic angiosarcoma
B wood dust and sinonasal carcinoma
C fungal α-amylase and asthma
D blue asbestos and lung cancer
E cadmium and renal failure

126. According to the 2003 British Thoracic Society/SIGN Guidelines on the Treatment of Asthma, step 3 following introduction of a short-acting β_2-agonist inhaler and regular low-dose inhaled steroids is:

A double dose of inhaled steroids
B add long-acting β_2-agonist
C add trial course of oral steroids
D add SR theophylline
E add leukotriene receptor antagonist (LTRA)

127–131. Using the British Hypertension Society 1999 Guidelines for Management of Hypertension, match the appropriate management option:

A Advise lifestyle changes and reassess monthly; treat if CHD risk > 15% over 10 years.
B Advise lifestyle changes, confirm within 4–12 weeks and treat if these values are sustained.
C Advise lifestyle changes, reassess weekly and treat if these values are sustained on repeat measurements over 4–12 weeks.
D Confirm over 3–4 weeks, then treat if these values are sustained.
E Confirm over 1–2 weeks, then treat if these values are sustained.
F Treat immediately.
G Admit to hospital for immediate treatment.

127. A 65-year-old man noted to have an initial BP of 220/100.

128. A 55-year-old woman is noted to have an initial BP of 170/100 but has no cardiovascular complications, end-organ damage or diabetes.

129. A 60-year-old man with NIDDM is noted to have a BP of 150/95.

130. A 45-year-old man with LVH is noted to have a BP of 180/105.

131. A 40-year-old obese healthy woman is noted to have a BP of 150/90.

132–137. Evidence-based management of hypertension

A calcium antagonist (dihydropyridine)
B thiazide diuretic
C ACE inhibitor
D angiotensin II receptor antagonists
E alpha-blocker
F calcium antagonists (rate-limiting)
G beta-blocker

For each of the patients below, select from the list of options above the **single** most appropriate antihypertensive drug, based on evidence:

132. A 75-year-old man with a history of gout is noted to have persistent BP > 170/80 over 3 months.

133. A 50-year-old Afro-Carribean man requires anti-hypertensive therapy.

134. A 70-year-old man with a history of prostatism has a persistent BP > 170/100.

135. A 55-year-old man has a history of heart failure and requires anti-hypertensive therapy.

136. A 60-year-old woman on ramipril complains of persistent tickly cough.

137. A 65-year-old man with a history of angina is noted to have persistently elevated BP.

138–140. Match the following gynaecological cancers with the relevant risk age group:

A carcinoma of the ovary
B cervical carcinoma
C vulval carcinoma
D carcinoma of the body of the uterus

138. Age group 20–64, with a median age of 52 years.

139. Over 40, with a median age of 60 years.

140. The majority occur in the 65–70 year age group.

141, 142. If the incidence of DVT in a high-risk population of women aged 35–45 on combined desogestrel and ethinyloestradiol is 10%, and the incidence of DVT is 5% in a similar population of women who do not use the combined oral contraceptive pill, then what are the values for:

141. Attributable risk?

    A 1%
    B 2%
    C 5%
    D 10%
    E 15%
    F 25%

142. Numbers needed to treat?

    A 10
    B 20
    C 25
    D 50
    E 100

143. Which of the following meningococcal vaccines is recommended for a family travelling to Saudi Arabia during the Hajj pilgrimage?

    A meningococcal group C
    B meningococcal group A
    C meningococcal group AC
    D meningococcal polysaccharide ACWY vaccine

144. The following symptoms may be associated with ricin (extract from beans of the castor oil plant):

    A cough
    B fever
    C bloody diarrhoea
    D seizure
    E heart failure

145–148. Interpret the following spirometry test results and match to the most likely diagnosis:

  A FEV1/FVC = 76% with an FEV1 of 2.5 l
  B FEV1/FVC = 82% with an FEV1 of 1 l
  C FEV1/FVC = 40% with an FEV1 of 1.5 l

145. Severe emphysema

146. Extrinsic allergic alveolitis

147. Asthma

148. Sarcoidosis

149. The initial treatment for acute anaphylaxis is:

  A 0.5 ml of 1 : 1000 adrenaline IM
  B 0.5 ml of 1 : 1000 adrenaline IV
  C 0.5 ml of 1 : 1000 adrenaline SC
  D 0.5 ml of 1 : 10,000 adrenaline IM
  E 0.5 ml of 1 : 10,000 adrenaline IV

150–153. Confidence intervals

Match the following statistical relevances with the confidence intervals depicted below:

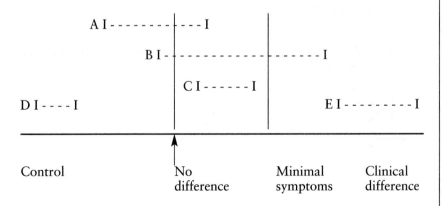

150. Statistically significant but with minimal symptoms.

151. Not statistically significant and may be harmful.

152. Statistically significant but not clinically significant.

153. Clinically significant.

154. If aspirin decreases the risk of cerebrovascular disease by 20% then what is the relative risk of cerebrovascular disease in users of aspirin versus non-users?

A 0.2
B 0.4
C 0.6
D 0.8
E 1.2

155. Relative risk is defined as:

A the incidence of disease in the non-exposed population divided by the incidence of disease in the exposed population
B the incidence of disease in the non-exposed population minus the incidence of disease in the exposed population
C the incidence of disease in the exposed population divided by the incidence of disease in the non-exposed population
D the incidence of disease in the exposed population minus the incidence of disease in the non-exposed population
E the incidence of disease in the general population

156. Initial treatment for allergic nasal polyps as recommended in the BNF is:

A Beconase nasal spray
B Betnesol nasal drops
C prednisolone
D xylometazoline nasal drops
E Rynacrom nasal spray

157. A 50-year-old woman is noted to have persistently elevated fasting blood glucose. She has a BMI of 31 and has tried to diet unsuccessfully. Which is the **single** most appropriate antidiabetic drug for her?

A oral sulfonylurea
B biguanide
C thiazolidinedione
D acarbose
E repaglinide

158. A 65-year-old woman presents with myalgia. The serum full blood count is normal and the ESR comes back as 40 mm/h. The next step should be:

A course of high-dose steroids, since she most likely has polymyalgia rheumatica
B arrange for CXR and AXR
C take blood for CRP, since it is more sensitive
D reassurance
E refer for temporal artery biopsy

159. The mother of an 8-year-old boy would like her son tested for allergy to peanuts, since it runs in the family. Which is the **single** most appropriate investigation?

A RAST
B serum allergen specific IgE
C skin prick test
D patch testing
E nasal smear

160. A 7-year-old boy presents with recurrent abdominal bloating, weight loss and diarrhoea. He is in the 5th percentile for height and weight. Which screening investigation is the **single** most sensitive?

A endomysial antibodies
B full blood count
C faecal fat estimation
D vitamin B_{12}/folate levels
E urea and electrolytes

161–164. Analgesia

A aspirin
B diamorphine
C diclofenac IM
D ibuprofen
E naratriptan
F paracetamol
G pizotifen
H tramadol PO

For each of the patients below, select from the list of options above the **single** most appropriate type of analgesia:

161. A 50-year-old man presents with vomiting and left loin pain. He has a history of renal stones.

162. A 55-year-old man presents with severe angina and a BP of 80/60.

163. A 60-year-old woman with metastatic breast cancer asks for analgesia for headaches.

164. A 30-year-old woman requests analgesia for migraines. She is on Prozac.

165. A 25-year-old woman states that she had her pill-free break but forgot to start a new pill pack on day 1. It is now day 2 and she has had UPSI yesterday. What is the **single** most appropriate management plan?

A Administer Levonelle-2.
B Offer an IUCD.
C Suggest she start the pack and omit the pill-free break.
D Wait until she sees her next period before starting the pill.
E Take 3 pills today and resume pack as normal tomorrow.

166. The following statements are true regarding the management of constipation in children:

A Rectal examination (PR) is often indicated to exclude faecal impaction.
B Abdominal x-ray must be obtained to exclude pathology.
C Lactulose may be prescribed.
D Evacuation of faecal impaction is offered under a GA.
E Faeces may be palpated in the abdomen.

167–171. Evidence-based management of LV dysfunction

A amlodipine
B diclofenac
C digoxin
D frusemide
E GTN
F losartan
G nicorandil
H nifedipine
I ramipril
J spironolactone
K verapamil
L warfarin

Match the scenarios below with the drugs listed above:

167. A 60-year-old man is noted to have LV dysfunction on echo and a history of angina. From the list above, which 2 drugs are most appropriate in his management?

168. Which 2 drugs are contraindicated with LV dysfunction?

169. A 70-year-old man is noted to have LV dysfunction on echo and has an irregularly irregular pulse rate. From the list above, which 2 drugs should be added to his management?

170. A 65-year-old man is noted to have LV dysfunction and has fluid overload. Which 2 drugs should be offered in his management?

171. A 55-year-old man with LV dysfunction continues to have fluid overload and now has sodium retention despite thiazide diuretic, ramipril and bisoprolol. What should be added next?

172. Diagnosis of diabetes mellitus is best made by:

A fasting blood glucose
B oral glucose tolerance test
C random blood glucose
D HbAIC
E capillary sample

173–177.

A acute lymphoblastic leukaemia
B acute myeloid leukaemia
C chronic granulocytic leukaemia
D chronic lymphocytic leukaemia
E non-Hodgkin lymphoma
F Hodgkin lymphoma
G iron-deficiency anaemia
H multiple myeloma
I sickle cell anaemia

For each of the patients below, select from the list of options above the **single** most likely diagnosis:

173. A 14-year-old male presents with recurrent gum bleeding, sore throat, mouth ulcers and malaise. On examination, he has a palpable spleen. Blood tests show elevated WCC with decreased platelets. Blood film shows a few blast cells. His father works in a gas station with regular exposure to petrol.

174. A 25-year-old female presents with an enlarged, painless cervical lymph node. She also reports drenching night sweats and has lost weight. Peripheral blood smear shows Reed–Sternberg cells with a bilobed, mirror-imaged nucleus.

175. A 70-year-old man presents with recurrent chest infections and chronic back pain. Blood tests reveal anaemia and elevated urea/creatinine. Blood tests reveal an elevated ESR and calcium. Bone marrow reveals an abundance of malignant plasma cells.

176. An 8-year-old boy presents with swelling of the hands and feet. Hb is 8 mg/dl. Peripheral blood smear reveals target cells and elongated crescent-shaped red blood cells.

177. A 65-year-old woman presents with dysphagia. She is also noted to have spoon-shaped fingernails and a smooth tongue. Blood smear reveals microcytic, hypochromic blood cells.

178–184. Algorithm for the management of jaundice

A conjugated
B unconjugated
C gallstones present
D no gallstones present
E CT scan
F ultrasound
G ERCP
H PTC
I liver biopsy

Complete the gaps in the algorithm from the list above:

JAUNDICE

History, examination, urine and blood tests including viral markers

Raised plasma (178) _____ BR   Raised plasma (179) _____ BR
Urinary urobilinogen increased   No urinary urobilinogen

(180) _____

No dilatation of common bile duct   Dilatation of common bile duct

(181) _____   (182) _____

If PTC or ERCP is normal,   (184) _____ or surgery
then (183) _____

185. A 20-year-old pregnant woman presents with asymptomatic bacteriuria. The most appropriate antibiotic regime is:

A cefadroxil 0.5–1 g bd × 3 days
B co-amoxiclavulanic acid 375 mg tds × 7 days
C nalidixic acid 1 g qds × 5 days
D nitrofurantoin 50 mg qds × 7 days
E trimethoprim 200 mg bd × 3 days

186. Risk factors for osteoporosis include:

A gastric surgery
B Muslim female
C repeated short courses of steroids
D overexercise
E smoking

187–190. Match the following age groups with the appropriate recommended immunizations. There may be more than one recommended vaccine per age group.

A adult DT
B polio
C MMR
D HiBDPT
E Men C

187. At 2, 3 and 4 months of age.

188. 12–15 months of age.

189. 3- to 4-year-olds (preschool).

190. 14- to 18-year-olds.

191–194. Urinary incontinence

    A vesicovaginal fistula
    B urinary tract infection
    C multiple sclerosis
    D disc prolapse
    E cystocoele
    F pelvic floor prolapse
    G senile vaginitis

For each of the patients below, select from the list of options above the **single** most likely diagnosis:

191. A 50-year-old woman reports constant urinary incontinence post hysterectomy.

192. A 55-year-old woman with a history of low back pain presents with altered sensation around the anus and urinary incontinence.

193. A 70-year-old woman reports 3 months of urinary incontinence. She is ashamed to bring this up with you. Coughing makes matters worse. MSU is normal.

194. A 40-year-old woman presents with double vision, weakness in both legs and urinary incontinence.

195–200. Childhood illnesses

    A appendicitis
    B bronchiolitis
    C gastroenteritis
    D hand, foot and mouth disease
    E Henoch–Schönlein purpura
    F Kawasaki's disease
    G meningitis
    H pneumonia

For each of the patients below, select from the list of options above the **single** most likely diagnosis.

195. A 13-year-old girl presents with a non-blanching rash and drowsiness.

196. A 10-year-old boy presents with a haemorrhagic purpuric rash over the lower half of his body.

197. An 8-year-old girl presents with fever, polymorphous rash, lip fissuring and erythema of the hands and feet.

198. An 18-month-old baby presents with fever and vomiting. The ears, throat and chest exams are normal.

199. A 2-month-old baby presents with wheeze and cough. On exam, basal creps are auscultated.

200. A 3-year-old girl presents with spiking fever, dry cough, left shoulder tip pain and left upper abdominal pain.

1. ABCDE Asplenia or severe dysfunction of the spleen (including homozygous sickle cell disease and coeliac syndrome), chronic heart disease, chronic liver disease (including cirrhosis), chronic lung disease, diabetes mellitus, chronic renal disease or nephrotic syndrome, and immunodeficiency or immunosuppression due to disease or treatment (including HIV at all stages) are all indications for pneumococcal vaccination. The MDA Agency Advice, August 2002, includes unvaccinated cochlear implant patients.

2. ABCDE Viagra is licensed for ED in men who have DM, MS, Parkinson's, poliomyelitis, prostate cancer, severe pelvic injury, spina bifida or spinal cord injury, or who have had radical pelvic surgery, prostatectomy or kidney transplant.

3. D

4. F

5. B

6. E

7. G

8. C At 6 months, a baby can sit with support, can transfer a cube from hand to hand and shows person preference.

9. E By 8 months, a baby can sit without support.

10. L A 5-year-old child can hop on one foot, can count 10–12 objects, knows 3–4 colours and shows friend preference.

11. A A 6-week baby can track an object 1 m away and smile and startle, and has both a Moro and a grasp reflex.

12. H   By 18 months, a baby can build a 3–4 cube tower, can speak 10–12 words, asks for a potty, can use a spoon and jumps with both feet.

13. K   A 4-year-old child can copy a circle and a cross, use a tricycle, catch a ball and knows its first and last names.

14. B   A 12-week-old baby can turn its head to sounds at the level of the ear. By 7 months, a baby can turn its head to sounds below the level of the ear.

15. A   However, if the driver was diagnosed with AIDS syndrome, revocation of the licence is recommended for group 2 entitlement.

16. H   Stable/unstable angina requires a cessation of driving if angina occurs at rest or at the wheel. For HGV drivers (group 2), revocation is recommended; however, relicensing can occur if the driver has been symptom-free for 6/52 and passes the exercise–stress test criteria.

17. D   A first fit associated with misuse of alcohol or drugs or a neurosurgical condition requires a ban on driving for at least 1 year, with medical review before restarting driving.

18. B

19. B   Any cerebrovascular condition (ie stroke due to TIA, amaurosis fugax or intracerebral haemorrhage) requires a ban on driving for at least 1 month. For group 2 entitlement, the ban is for 1 year.

20. C   Current recommendations suggest permethrin or malathion as first-line treatment for scabies. Hot baths have now been found to increase absorption of topical treatment into the bloodstream away from the site of action, ie the skin. All members of the affected household should be treated.

21. E

22. A

23. B

24. C

25. F

26. H

27. F

28. D

29. C

30. A

31. G

32. B

33. C

34. B

35. F

36. I

37. D

38. J

39. H

40. A

41. ABCDE

42. B

43. ABCE   Urgent referral is recommended for painless macroscopic haematuria in adults.

44. ABCDE

45. C

46. E

47. D

48. C

49. F

50. E

51. A   These symptoms warrant an MRI of the internal acoustic meati to exclude acoustic neuroma.

52. D

53. B

54. C

55. E

56. A

57. C

58. D

59. G

60. A

61. F

62. E

63. ABCD   Domiciliary oxygen is recommended for patients with pulmonary malignancy or other terminal disease with disabling dyspnoea.

64. ABCDEF   Pregnant women should avoid basil, cedarwood, clary sage, juniper berry, marjoram, myrrh and sage. Patients with epilepsy should avoid fennel, sage and rosemary. Hypertensive patients should avoid rosemary, sage, thyme and stimulating spice oils. Citrus oils and bergamot should be avoided prior to sun exposure. Patients using homeopathy should then avoid camphor, chamomile and mint oils, since these may neutralize the effects of homeopathy, and finally skin testing should be performed to assess allergy or skin irritation.

65. A

66. ABCD

67. B

68. C

69. A

70. E

71. D

72. F

73. D

74. B

75. A

76. E

77. F

78. C

79. E

80. B

81. A

82. H

83. B

84. D   Six weeks is advised to allow the baby's liver enzymes to mature.

85. F

86. D

87. B

88. B

89. C

90. F

91. G

92. J

93. L

94. N

95. M

96. H

97. C

98. A

99. B

100. D

101. F

102. A   Items of service payments include night visits, emergency treatment, immediately necessary treatment, cervical cytology fee, contraceptive fee, anaesthetic fee, dental haemorrhage fee, health promotion fees, immunizations, maternity fees and minor op fees.

103. A

104. C   Practice allowances include absence allowances to cover locums, study leave, PGEA course, confinement, etc., assistant or associate's allowances, basic and initial practice allowances, designated area allowance and rural practice payment.

105. B Reimbursement includes GO computer reimbursement scheme, dispensing fees, out-of-hours development scheme, practice staff scheme, and reimbursement of rent, rate and sewerage.

106. C

107. A

108. A

109. D Private medical work includes reports for insurance companies, solicitors, lecturing, fitness to drive, HGV licence, court witness, cremation fees and other private medical exams.

110. E Capitation fees include standard capitation fee for patients aged <65, 65–74 and 75 and over, child health surveillance, deprivation payments, registration fee, and temporary resident fees.

111. C

112. D

113. E

114. B

115. A All squints require ophthamological assessment. Management is divided into the 3 'O's : optical, orthoptic and operation. The refractive state of the eyes is determined after use of mydriatic eye drops, and the eyes are inspected to exclude cataract, macular scarring, optic atrophy, retinoblastoma etc. Spectacles are offered to correct any refractive errors. Orthoptic is the patching of the good eye to encourage use of the squinting (lazy) eye. Finally, resection and recession of the rectus muscles is reserved for cosmesis or alignment.

116. B

117. G

118. C

119. A

120. K

121. D

122. I

123. H

124. J

125. ABCDE   Commercial bakers are exposed to fungal amylase additives to flour, which cause occupational asthma. Cadmium is also associated with respiratory disease.

126. B   Guidelines have recently been changed as of February 2003. The addition of long-acting β_2-agonists is now advocated, prior to increasing the dose of inhaled steroids to 800 μg/day. If there is no response to an inhaled LABA plus increased steroid, then an LTRA or SR theophylline is introduced. Step 4 is as before, increasing the inhaled steroids to 2000 μg/day and possibly adding an LTRA. Step 5 is the introduction of daily oral steroids and referral of the patient for specialist care.

127. F

128. C

129. B

130. D

131. A

132. A

133. B

134. E

135. C

136. D

137. G

138. B   Cervical cancer is the second most common malignancy after breast cancer.

139. D   Carcinoma of the body of the uterus is less frequent than cancer of the cervix or ovary.

140. C

141. C   Attributable risk is the incidence in the exposed population minus the incidence in the non-exposed population.

142. B   NNT=1/ARR%= 1/ (% treated group with desired outcome minus % controls with desired outcome).

143. D   35 deaths occurred during the Hajj pilgrimage of 2001, with >100 cases of W135 serotype meningococcal meningitis. In 2004, the Hajj will take place in the third week of January. Outside the Hajj and Umrah pilgrimages, Men A&C vaccination is adequate and also recommended from travel in other areas of risk, ie Nepal, Pakistan, Bhutan and the meningitis belt of Africa.

144. ABCDE   Ricin is 6000 times more lethal than cyanide per gram. There is no cure and treatment is supportive. Symptoms may surface between 1 and 7 days following exposure by inhalation, ingestion or injection. Ingestion of 8 castor oil seeds is lethal in an adult.

145. C In obstructive disease, the FEV1/FVC ratio is < 80% with an FEV1 of < 80% predicted. In restrictive disease, the FEV1/FVC ratio is > 80% with an FEV1 of < 80% predicted. Normally, the FEV1 should be > 80% predicted with an FEV1/FVC ratio between 70% and 80%.

146. B

147. A

148. B

149. A

150. B

151. A

152. C

153. E

154. D The relative risk in this case is calculated as 1− (20% of 1) = 0.8.

155. C Option D is the definition of attributable risk and option E the definition of absolute risk. Know how to calculate relative risk and NNR for the exam (popular question).

156. B

157. B

158. D The upper limits of normal for ESR = (10 + age) divided by 2. This women's ESR is normal, but you may wish to repeat in 6 months. Alarm bells should ring if the ESR is > 100 mm/h. Causes of elevated ESR include rheumatoid arthritis, infection, malignancy, connective tissue disorders (giant cell arteritis), sarcoidosis and renal disease.

159. C   Skin prick testing should be conducted in a specialist chest clinic, since there is a high risk of anaphylaxis.

160. A

161. C

162. B   Although you would also give aspirin while awaiting the ambulance.

163. H

164. E

165. C

166. CDE   It is rare to subject a child to a PR examination. Firm stool should be palpable during abdominal examination.

167. AE

168. BK

169. CL

170. DI

171. J

172. A   An FBG > 7 confirms diabetes. If the FBG is borderline (between 7 and 8), do an oral glucose tolerance test. The OGTT should normally be < 7.8 at 2 hours postprandial.

173. A

174. F

175. H

176. I

177. G

178. B

179. A

180. F

181. D

182. C

183. I

184. G

185. A   50% of *E. coli* are now resistant to ampicillin.

186. ABCE   Other risk factors include excessive alcohol, repeated steroid use in inflammatory bowel disease, family history, inactivity, lack of oestrogen, and low testosterone in men.

187. BDE

188. C

189. CD

190. AB

191. A

192. D

193. F

194. C

195. A

196. E

197. F

198. C

199. B

200. H   Left-sided basal pneumonia can present in children with left-sided abdominal pain with referred shoulder tip pain from irritation of the diaphragm via the phrenic nerve.

1–5. Match the following antihypertensive drugs with their noted side-effects. There may be more than one answer:

A beta-blocker
B diuretic
C ACE inhibitor
D angiotensin receptor antagonist
E calcium antagonist
F alpha-blocker

1. Cold hands and feet

2. Stress incontinence

3. Headache

4. Flushing

5. Impotence

6. The following statements are TRUE concerning case–control studies:

A They can prove causation.
B They cannot calculate risk ratio.
C They are particularly useful for investigating rare diseases.
D They are expensive to conduct.
E They are retrospective.

7. A 60-year-old woman sustains a hip fracture. Upon discharge from hospital, you decide to put her on medication for osteoporosis. Besides Calcichew D3 Forte, you should add (single best answer):

A calcitonin
B raloxifene
C HRT
D alendronic acid
E tiludronic acid

8. Contraindications to the use of nicotine replacement therapy include which of the following (multiple best answer)?

A breastfeeding
B severe cardiovascular disease
C recent TIA
D chronic psoriasis
E diabetes mellitus

9. Which three statements are true concerning anthrax?

A It is a notifiable disease.
B Contacts of exposed individuals require prophylaxis.
C ID50 is the dose required to infect 50% of exposed individuals.
D CXR findings are classic for anthrax.
E Ciprofloxacin is the antibiotic of choice.

10. Which of the following diseases are notifiable to the Consultant in Communicable Disease Control (multiple best answer)?

A cholera
B food poisoning
C measles
D scarlet fever
E viral hepatitis

11. A 1-year-old child presents with a history of 12 hours of right earache and high fever. On exam, $T = 39°C$ and the tympanic membrane is red and bulging. The most appropriate treatment is (single best answer):

A ibuprofen
B amoxicillin
C trimethoprim
D Calpol
E reassurance and review

12. The following statements are TRUE regarding coronary heart disease and air travel:

A There need be no bar with unstable angina.
B A symptom-free patient following coronary angioplasty is fit to travel after 2 weeks.
C If a patient with coronary heart disease cannot manage a flight of stairs without stopping, he is not fit for flying.
D Travel should be delayed for 3 weeks following a recent myocardial infarction.
E If a patient with LVF requires oxygen at rest, flying is contraindicated.

13. The **single** most common presentation of stroke is:

    A sudden visual field deficit
    B sudden onset of hemiplegia
    C dysphagia
    D loss of consciousness
    E aphasia

14. The following statements are TRUE regarding evidence-based management of stroke (multiple best answer):

    A Aspirin 300 mg should be started within 48 hours of a
      haemorrhagic stroke.
    B Thombolysis is offered routinely.
    C Heparin prophylaxis is indicated if the patient has morbid obesity.
    D Heparin is indicated for recurrent embolic TIAs.
    E DVT and PE develop in 50% of patients after an ischaemic stroke.

15–19. Statin trials

    A AFCAPS/TexCaps, *JAMA*
    B CARE, *NEJM*, 1996
    C 4S Trial, *Lancet* 1994
    D Heart protection study, *Lancet* 2002
    E WOSCOPS
    F LIPID study, *NEJM* 1998

    Match the following study descriptions with their correlating trials
    listed above:

15. This study showed the benefits of reducing cholesterol in healthy
    men and women with average cholesterol levels.

16. This 5-year, randomized controlled study of 20,536 individuals
    with cardiac disease or diabetes showed that 40 mg of simvastatin
    reduced the risk of MI, stroke and revascularization by one-third,
    even in patients with normal or low blood cholesterol levels.

17. This was a prospective trial of 4,444 patients with coronary heart
    disease and raised cholesterol. This trial showed a reduction of rel-
    ative risk of coronary mortality of 42% in patients treated with
    simvastatin 20–40 mg a day. Greatest benefit was achieved in
    patients > 60 years of age or patients with DM.

18. This randomized trial of 6,595 middle-aged men with a mean cholesterol of 7 mmol/l showed a 31% reduction in coronary mortality in those treated with 40 mg pravastatin a day and a 20% reduction in cholesterol in the treated group.

19. In this randomized controlled trial, 4,159 men and women aged 21–75 years who had suffered an MI in the past 2 years and had an average total cholesterol of 5.4 mmol/l were randomized to pravastatin or placebo and followed at 5 years. The study showed that reducing cholesterol level with pravastatin after MI reduced risk of CHD death/non-fatal MI by 24%, of fatal MI by 37% and of stroke by 28%.

20. The following statements are TRUE concerning renal medicine:

   A Patients with type I diabetes and repeated microalbuminuria should be commenced on an ACE inhibitor.
   B Patients with a serum creatinine > 150 µmol/l should be referred to a nephrologist.
   C Renal function should be checked at initiation and 2–3 weeks after starting or increasing an ACE inhibitor or angiotensin receptor II inhibitor.
   D Orthostatic proteinuria in an adolescent with a total daily protein excretion of < 1 g may be ignored.
   E Patients younger than 40 with microscopic haematuria and hypertension should be referred to a nephrologist.

21. The following statements are TRUE concerning drug therapy for obesity:

   A Orlistat acts by inhibiting the action of pancreatic lipase, thus reducing the digestion and absorption of dietary fat.
   B According to NICE guidelines, patients must have a BMI > 30 kg/m^2 and must have produced a weight loss > 2.5 kg over 4 weeks before commencing orlistat.
   C Blood pressure and pulse must be monitored frequently prior and during treatment with orlistat.
   D Sibutramine acts by promoting and prolonging satiety after eating.
   E Side-effects of sibutramine include fatty oily stool.

22–25. Orthopaedic conditions

A plantar fasciitis
B patello-femoral syndrome
C patella tendonitis
D Osgood–Schlatter disease
E calcaneal stress fracture

For each of the patients below, select from the list of options above the **single** most likely diagnosis:

22. A 40-year-old woman complains of heel pain. Pain is worse putting the heel on to the floor in the morning but eases as she walks. On examination, she has point tenderness 4 cm forward from the heel.

23. A 20-year-old woman presents with heel pain. She enjoys running in marathons. Pain is elicited on squeezing the lateral aspect of the calcaneus.

24. A 25-year-old ballet dancer reports anterior knee pain with clicking and crepitus of the knee. On examination, she has medial patellar tenderness and a mild effusion.

25. A 14-year-old girl reports anterior knee pain. On examination, the tibial tubercle is prominent and tender.

26–31. Eye conditions

A acute conjunctivitis
B acute iritis
C central retinal artery occlusion
D central retinal vein occlusion
E closed angled glaucoma
F posterior communicating aneurysm
G retinal detachment
H vitreous haemorrhage

26. An 8-year-old child presents with sudden diplopia, ptosis and a lateral diverging eye.

27. A 60-year-old woman c/o a 'curtain coming down' over her right eye with painless loss of vision. She mentions seeing flashing lights first.

28. A 40-year-old man c/o a painful red eye with photophobia and pain on accommodation. The pupil is irregular.

29. A 70-year-old woman presents with a cloudy cornea, reduced visual acuity and painful red eye.

30. A 75-year-old woman presents with sudden loss of vision in the left eye with acuity reduced to finger counting. The fundus resembles a bloodstorm!

31. A 60-year-old woman presents with sudden loss of vision in the right eye with acuity reduced to light perception. The retina appears white with a cherry-red spot on the macula. She comments that she had transient blindness before full blindness of the right eye.

32–34. ECGs

    A acute myocardial infarction
    B acute pericarditis
    C pulmonary embolus

Match the following descriptions of ECG abnormalities with the correct diagnosis from the list above:

32. Q-waves in leads II, III, avF with ST-elevation and T-wave inversion.

33. Deep S-waves in lead I, pathological Q-waves in III and inverted T-wave in lead III.

34. Concave, saddle-shaped ST-segment elevation.

35. The following statements are TRUE concerning heart failure:

    A NICE recommendations 2003 suggest GPs use a blood test for the marker N-terminal pro-brain natriuretic peptide (NT-proBNP) to exclude heart failure.
    B Echocardiogram is the gold standard for diagnosing heart failure.
    C Angiotensin receptor blockers are a first-line therapy in chronic heart failure.
    D Spironolactone should be added to patients in advanced heart failure (NYHA class III/IV).
    E Beta-blockers are associated with deterioration in the patient's quality of life during the first 3 months of therapy.

36. Which of the following should be suggested for a baby with intractable colic (single best answer)?

    A soya milk
    B sugared water
    C anticholinergic drugs
    D Infacol
    E gripe water

37–42. Laboratory investigations

    A ESR
    B ferritin
    C platelets
    D serum protein electrophoresis
    E vitamin B_{12}
    F white blood count

For each of the patients below, select from the list of options above the **single** most discriminating investigation:

37. A 40-year-old man post gastrectomy presents with anaemia.

38. A 30-year-old woman with a history of fibroids presents with angular cheilosis.

39. A 20-year-old woman presents with recurrent epistaxis, easy bruisability and heavy periods.

40. A 35-year-old man presents with chronic fatigue and shortness of breath with mild exertion. He is also noted to have bronzed skin and arthralgia of the MCP joints.

41. A 10-year-old boy presents with a purple rash on his buttocks, which does not disappear on pressure.

42. A 70-year-old man presents with a compression fracture of his spine.

43. According to the NICE guidelines for the management of type 2 diabetes, the following statements are TRUE:

A Patients with type 2 diabetes should be tested annually for microalbuminuria.
B Patients with type 2 diabetes should have annual serum fasting lipids.
C Patients who do not have manifest cardiovascular disease should have their heart disease risk estimated annually.
D Patients whose blood pressure is found to be > 160/100 mmHg should be treated with ACE inhibitors.
E Aim for blood pressure < 140/80 mmHg.

44. According to evidence-based medicine, the **single** most appropriate step to take in the management of a male patient noted to have a total cholesterol of 6.0 mmol/l, LDL-C of 3.5 mmol/l and TG of 2 mmol/l is:

A Commence statin 40 mg nocte.
B Offer dietary advice.
C Assess coronary heart disease risk.
D Refer to specialist lipid clinic.
E Commence fibrate.

45. A 50-year-old woman reports night sweats and hot flushes. Which blood test would you order to confirm menopause?

A FSH
B LH
C progesterone
D prolactin
E testosterone

46. The Royal College of Physicians suggest that bone mineral density measurements should be offered to the following groups of patients:

A radiographic evidence of vertebral deformity
B body mass index < 19 kg/m^2
C prednisolone > 7.5 mg daily for 6 months or more
D premature menopause (age < 45 years)
E maternal history of hip fracture

47. An 8-year-old girl presents with 3 days of fever, sore throat and generalized lymphadenopathy. FBC reveals raised WCC, mostly atypical lymphocytes and mildly elevated ALT. Monospot test comes back as negative. The most appropriate step is:

    A Arrange for immunofluorescence test for EBV-specific IgM.
    B Repeat monospot test.
    C Reassure patient that she does not have glandular fever.
    D Arrange for liver scan.
    E Take throat swab for streptococcus.

48. The **single** most appropriate treatment for senile watery rhinorrhoea is:

    A sympathomimetic drug, ie pseudoephedrine
    B topical nasal ipratropium spray, ie Rinatec
    C topical antihistamine nasal spray, ie Rhinolast
    D Betnesol nasal drops
    E sodium cromoglycate

49. Recognized treatments for nasal polyps include all of the following **except**:

    A functional endoscopic sinus surgery (FESS)
    B snare polypectomy
    C Betnesol nasal drops
    D oral corticosteroids
    E topical nasal ipratropium spray

50. Recognized treatments of severe symptomatic pulmonary hypertension include:

    A calcium channel blockers
    B prostacyclin (Epoprostenol) infusion
    C regular nebulization of Iloprost
    D Bosentan (orally active non-selective antagonist of endothelin)
    E heart–lung transplantation

51. Select the **single** most appropriate drug for treatment of depression in the elderly:

    A donepezil
    B dothiepin
    C moclobemide
    D sertraline
    E venlafaxine

52. A 40-year-old mature student is diagnosed with schizophrenia. His acute psychosis is managed in hospital. Upon discharge, he should be maintained on:

A clozapine
B haloperidol
C olanzapine
D piportal
E risperidone

53–57. Urinanalysis

A RBC > 300/mm³, WBC 100/mm³, no organisms
B RBC 100/mm³, WBC 100/mm³, no organisms
C RBC 50/mm³, WBC < 10/mm³, no organisms
D RBC < 10/mm³, WBC 100/mm³, *E. coli* growth, urine specific gravity 1.025
E no RBCs, no WBC, urine specific gravity 1.002

Match the urinanalysis reports with the single most likely diagnosis from the list below:

53. Acute pyelonephritis.

54. Transitional cell carcinoma of the bladder.

55. Diabetes insipidus.

56. Renal calculus.

57. Renal tuberculosis.

58. Select **two** best answers for the treatment of scabies:

A Wash all bedding in boiling water.
B Wash curtains and steam-clean carpets.
C Hot bath before treatment application.
D Treat all members of the household.
E Apply cream twice, 1 week apart.

59. Select **two** correct statements regarding the spread and treatment of clothing lice:

   A It can walk from person to person.
   B Wash clothes in water > 60°C.
   C Lives on the hair and body.
   D Requires treatment with insecticides.
   E Lice can survive if clothes are not worn for 3 days or more.

60–65. Contraception
   A IUCD
   B Mirena
   C Levonelle-2
   D Depo-Provera injections
   E POP
   F combined oral contraceptive
   G condom
   H norethisterone
   I lactational amenorrhoea method (LAM)
   J sterilization

   For each of the patients below, select from the list of options above the **single** most appropriate form of contraception:

60. A 40-year-old woman with a history of menorrhagia requests contraception. She is forgetful, very busy and hates needles. She does not plan on having any more children.

61. A 20-year-old woman requests contraception. She had UPSI on day 12 of her cycle, which was 2 days ago. She was not on any form of contraception.

62. A 30-year-old woman requests a pill to help her stop her periods while she is holidaying in Corsica.

63. A 32-year-old woman with a history of polycystic ovarian disease requests contraception.

64. A 25-year-old woman with multiple sexual partners requests contraception. She smokes 40 cigarettes a day and her BMI is > 30. She has had 2 abortions in the past.

65. A 30-year-old woman 4 weeks postpartum requests contraception. She is breastfeeding and has not had a period.

66–70. Analgesia

A bisphosphonates
B NSAIDs
C COX-2 inhibitors
D tramadol
E methotrexate
F local steroid injection
G Futuro splint

For each of the patients below, select from the list of options above the **single** most appropriate form of analgesia.

66. A 25-year-old pregnant woman complains of numbness and tingling in the thumb, index and middle fingers of her right hand that is worse at night.

67. A 50-year-old woman with metastatic breast carcinoma complains of headaches.

68. A 55-year-old woman presents with a hot and swollen MT joint. She has had no relief with paracetamol. She has no history of peptic ulcer disease.

69. A 65-year-old woman suffers from disabling rheumatoid arthritis of the hands, wrists and right knee. She also has active peptic ulcer disease and heart failure.

70. A 40-year-old carpenter presents with pain on the lateral aspect of his elbow. He reports that the pain is worse when he uses his screwdriver. You suspect tennis elbow.

71. The **single** best cleaning agent for spilled vomit on the surgery floor is:

A Betadine
B chlorhexidine
C hypochlorite
D sodium chloride
E sodium perborate

72. A 30-year-old woman is found to have positive antiphospholipid antibody following a first-trimester miscarriage. She is at risk of:

    A arterial thrombosis
    B deep venous thrombosis
    C multi-infarct dementia
    D preeclampsia
    E stroke

73. Which of the following scenarios suggest urgent referral to a specialist breast clinic (single best answer)?

    A A 28-year-old woman on the COC reports tender, lumpy breasts.
    B A 40-year-old woman reports moderate breast pain but no discrete palpable lesion.
    C A 45-year-old woman reports nipple discharge from 2 ducts that is not bloodstained.
    D A 35-year-old breastfeeding woman reports persistent signs of sepsis in her left breast.
    E A 32-year-old woman presents with localized persistent nodularity in her right breast.

74–77. Investigations for jaundice

    A ERCP
    B liver biopsy
    C liver ultrasound
    D percutaneous transhepatic cholangiography
    E serum antimitochondrial antibodies
    F viral serology

For each of the patients below, select from the list of options above the **single** most discriminating investigation:

74. A 30-year-old businessman returns from a trip to the Far East and complains of anorexia, malaise, pale stools and dark urine.

75. A 45-year-old woman presents with a 3-year history of jaundice, pruritis, pale stools and dark urine.

76. A 40-year-old man presents with jaundice and malaise. His ferritin level is high and his LFTs are mildly elevated. He does not drink alcohol.

77. A 60-year-old man presents with jaundice, pale stools and dark urine following laparoscopic cholecystectomy. Ultrasound reveals dilated common bile duct.

78–83. Respiratory conditions

A amoxicillin
B clarithromycin
C losartan
D prednisolone
E ramipril
F salbutamol inhaler

For each of the patients below, select from the list of options above the **single** most appropriate treatment option:

78. A 50-year-old farmer presents with sudden onset of dry cough, fever and shortness of breath. Chest exam reveals basal crackles.

79. A 55-year-old man on bendrofluazide for hypertension now presents with cough, orthopnoea and paroxysmal nocturnal dyspnoea. Chest examination reveals basal rales.

80. A 30-year-old man presents with nocturnal cough. His FEV1 is 70% of predicted.

81. A 20-year-old man presents with swinging fever, non-productive cough and tender subcutaneous nodules on his anterior legs.

82. A 60-year-old woman on ramipril develops a tickly cough. Chest exam is normal.

83. A 50-year-old homeless man smelling of alcohol presents with fever and a productive cough. Chest exam reveals coarse rhonchi.

84–90. Fitness to drive

A no driving licence restrictions
B 1 month off driving
C 6 months off driving
E 12 months off driving
F disqualifies from driving until treated
G permanently barred and requires DVLA notification
H refusal or revocation
I driving must cease until cause identified
J relicensing when symptom-free for 6/52

Match the following scenarios with the appropriate fitness-to-drive regulations:

84. A man reaches his 70th birthday and denies medical disability.

85. A 50-year-old red-bus driver has a persistent BP of 180/100 mmHg.

86. A 60-year-old man is diagnosed with metastatic carcinoma of the lung with secondaries in the bone and brain.

87. A 40-year-old man has an acute subdural haematoma requiring burr holes to evacuate.

88. A 30-year-old man has colour blindness and a visual acuity of 6/9 in both eyes.

89. A 20-year-old IVDA heroin misuser tests positive for opiates in his urine. He would like to initiate methadone treatment.

90. A 35-year-old HGV driver reports that he fainted at the sight of the birth of his first child.

91–95. Glomerulopathy

A IgA nephropathy
B minimal change glomerulonephritis
C Henoch–Schönlein purpura
D thin membrane nephropathy
E focal segmental glomerulosclerosis
F mesangiocapillary glomerulonephritis
G membranous nephropathy
H proliferative GN
I rapidly progressive GN

For each of the patients below, select from the list of options above the **single** most likely diagnosis:

91. A 4-year-old boy presents with proteinuria, oedema and hypoalbuminuria. Renal biopsy shows fusion of podocytes on electron microscopy.

92. A 20-year-old man with HIV presents with nephrotic syndrome and hypertension. Renal biopsy shows hyalinization of glomerular capillaries and positive IF for IgM and C3.

93. A 35-year-old woman with SLE presents with renal impairment. Renal biopsy reveals thickened BM, IF positive for IgG and C3, and subepithelial deposits on EM.

94. An 80-year-old woman presents with loin pain, haematuria and fever. She was well a month prior. Her ESR is elevated and she has fundoscopic features of giant cell arteritis. Renal biopsy reveals a focal necrotizing GN with crescent formation.

95. A 10-year-old boy with sickle cell disease presents with features of nephrotic syndrome. Renal biopsy reveals large glomeruli with double BM and subendothelial deposits.

96. The following statements are correct regarding recent evidence on HRT (multiple best answer):

   A According to the WHI (Women's Health Initiative) study, for every 10,000 person-years there were seven more CHD events and eight more strokes than in the non-HRT group.
   B According to the HERS (Heart and Estrogen/Progestin Replacement Study), the absolute risk for VTE per 100,000 women per year was 620 in HRT users and 230 in non HRT users.
   C Women taking sequential HRT for more than 1 year are considered at higher risk of developing endometrial cancer.
   D The risk of breast cancer is equal to non-users after 5 years off HRT.
   E Raloxifene is useful in the management of menopausal symptoms.

97. The following drugs are recommended for the management of mild benign prostatic hypertrophy (multiple best answer):

   A cyproterone acetate
   B finasteride
   C indoramin
   D terazosin
   E tolterodine tartrate

98–102. Groin lumps

   A direct inguinal hernia
   B femoral hernia
   C incarcerated hernia
   D indirect inguinal hernia
   E psoas abscess
   F saphena varix

   For each of the clinical examination findings below, select from the list of options above the single most likely diagnosis:

98. A small lump is palpated in the groin medially. It transmits a cough impulse. It disappears when the patient lies down.

99. A lump arising in the superficial inguinal canal is felt on your fingertip when the patient coughs.

100. A lump arising in the superficial inguinal canal is felt against the pulp of your finger when the patient coughs.

101. A fluctant mass is palpated in the groin of an indigent. He also c/o back pain and is found to have a swinging pyrexia.

102. A 35-year-old woman presents with a mass above the inguinal liga-ment pointing downwards to the thigh. The lump is felt below and lateral to the pubic tubercle.

103–106. Immunological investigations

A antimitochondrial antibody
B antineutrophil cytoplasmic antibody
C antinuclear antibody
D antiphospholipid antibody
E antibody to reticulin
F rheumatoid factor
G thyroid antibodies

For each of the patients below, select from the list of options above the single most discriminating investigation:

103. A 40-year-old woman presents with a photosensitive malar rash over both cheeks and the bridge of her nose and chronic muscu-loskeletal pain.

104. A 30-year-old woman presents with 3 recurrent miscarriages. She also suffers from chronic migraines.

105. A 40-year-old woman presents with itching, jaundice and upper GI bleed.

106. A 60-year-old man presents with recurrent epistaxis, hypertension and microscopic haematuria.

107–112. Evidence-based treatment of metastatic breast carcinoma

    A aminoglutethimide
    B high-dose chemotherapy
    C megestrol
    D paclitaxel
    E radiotherapy
    F standard-dose chemotherapy
    G stilboestrol
    H tamoxifen
    I trilostane

For each of the conditions below, select from the list of options above the **single** most appropriate treatment option, based on evidence:

107. First-line therapy for estrogen receptor-positive widespread carcinoma.

108. Bony metatastases.

109. For relapse on tamoxifen.

110. Does not improve survival in patients who have undergone standard-dose chemotherapy.

111. Is recommended by NICE for the treatment of advanced breast cancer where initial cytotoxic chemotherapy has failed or is inappropriate.

112. Is tolerated with a PPI and corticosteroids.

113. Which of the following methods may be used for management of scars?

    A acrylic casts
    B intralesional corticosteroid injection
    C laser therapy
    D silicone sheeting
    E static splints

114–116. Red Book

A basic practice
B capitation
C cost
D initial practice
E notional

For each of the numbered gaps, choose one word from the list above that best completes the sentence. Each option may be used once, more than once or not at all.

A practitioner building a new separate purpose-built premises may be reimbursed a (114) _____ rent. A pre-agreed percentage of the total cost of the building is reimbursed to the practitioner each year. Owner-occupiers are paid (115) _____ rent allowance for allowing use of their private building for NHS purposes. The rent payment is based on the current market rent value assessed by the district valuer. New partners are expected to buy into the practice if the allowance is based on (116) _____ rent.

117. According to Groves' classification, the different types of heart-sink patients are?

A aggressive manipulators
B entitled demanders
C dependent clingers
D manipulative help-rejectors
E self-destructive deniers

118. Exceptions to generic prescribing include:

A anticonvulsants
B ciclosporin
C diltiazem
D nifedipine
E theophylline

119. Deaths that need to be reported to the coroner include:

A infant deaths
B death through neglect
C death due to industrial disease
D deceased not attended by a doctor in their last illness
E deceased not seen by the doctor completing the death certificate after death

120. The following substances have been shown to cause occupational asthma:

A flour
B glutaraldehyde
C isocyanate
D lead
E nickel

121–125. Childhood rashes

A chickenpox
B erythema multiforme
C erythema nodosum
D Kawasaki's disease
E hand, foot and mouth disease
F herpes simplex
G measles
H molluscum contagiosum
I scarlet fever

For each of the patients below, select from the list of options above the single most likely diagnosis:

121. A 10-year-old boy presents with three pale umbilicated papules on his neck. He enjoys swimming at school.

122. A 3-year-old girl presents with painful mouth ulcers and red spots on her palms. She is not unwell.

123. A 15-year-old girl presents with crops of pale erythematous–violaceous macules surrounded by concentric rings on her palms. She had taken a course of penicillin.

124. A 2-year-old boy presents with high fever and a morbilliform rash which started over his forehead and cheeks and has now spread to his trunk and limbs. He has a hoarse cough and his mouth is painful and red.

125. A 7-year-old boy presents with a sore throat and a truncal rash of pink coalescent rings. He has a strawberry tongue.

126. Which of the following are examples of longitudinal studies?

   A case–control studies
   B cohort studies
   C prevalence studies
   D prospective studies
   E retrospective studies

127. Factors influencing predicted normal lung function values include:

   A age
   B ethnic origin
   C height
   D sex
   E weight

128. The **single** best treatment for scalp ringworm in children is:

   A clotrimazole cream
   B ketoconazole shampoo
   C oral griseofulvin
   D oral itraconazole
   E terbinafine cream

129. The following are recognized treatments for cradle cap:

   A arachis oil
   B Betadine shampoo
   C Capasal shampoo
   D Cocois scalp ointment
   E olive oil

130. Which **two** statements regarding treatment for migraines are true?

   A $5HT_1$ antagonists are useful in the treatment of acute attacks.
   B Ergot alkaloids may be prescribed prophylactically.
   C Ismethoptene mucate in combination with paracetamol is licensed for the treatment of migraines.
   D Beta-blockers may be used for migraine prophylaxis.
   E Pizotifen may be used for treatment of acute attacks.

131–141. Evidence-based management of anaemia

    A anaemia of chronic disease
    B assess iron status
    C blood film
    D B_{12}
    E beta- or alpha-thalassaemia trait
    F DAT reticulocyte count
    G ESR
    H Hb electrophoresis
    I history of diet, drugs and alcohol
    J iron deficiency anaemia
    K LFTs

For each of the numbered gaps, choose one word from the above list.

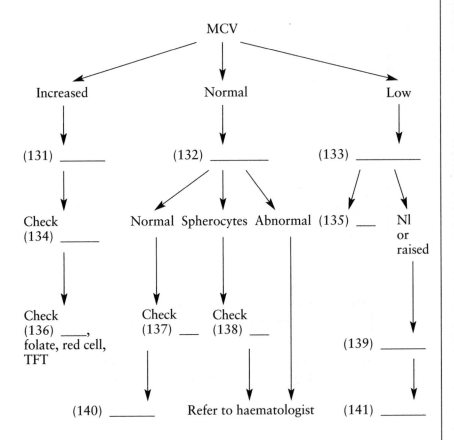

142. A 70-year-old woman presents with swollen lower legs. She is on 5 mg of felodipine for hypertension and indomethacin for rheumatic disease. Her BP is currently 140/70. The **single** most appropriate step is:

A to prescribe elastic stockings
B to add a thiazide diuretic
C to change felodipine to an ACE inhibitor
D to add a loop diuretic
E to change indomethacin to a COX-2 inhibitor

143. A 30-year-old woman complains of headaches, feeling TAT and disoriented. She reports that she moved into a council flat in November. The flat is damp with visible mould. She also suffers from asthma and is on Dianette for contraception. The **single** most appropriate management would be:

A Increase inhalers since patient is allergic to mould.
B Change Dianette to POP.
C Advise patient to test for carbon monoxide poisoning.
D Arrange patch testing for mould sensitization.
E Prescribe antidepressant.

144–150. Welfare Benefits

Match the following allowances with their correct descriptions:

A Attendance Allowance
B Disabled Concessions
C Disability Living Allowance
D Disability Working Allowance
E Incapacity Benefits
F Income Support
G Invalid Care Allowance
H Severe Disability Allowance
I Social Fund Benefits
J Unemployment Benefit

144. A tax-free, non-means-tested allowance for a person over the age of 65 with a severe physical or mental disability requiring care during the day or day and night.

145. An allowance for a person aged between 18 and 65 with 80% or greater disability who is unable to work for 28 weeks. NI contributions are not mandatory.

146. A tax-free but income-related and means-tested allowance for a person on low income who is older than 16 and works at least 16 hours a week and is receiving one of the disability allowances.

147. This is paid at 3 different rates (short-term at lower rate, short-term at higher rate and long-term after 1 year) to a person unfit for work on medical grounds for > 28 weeks and who has paid NI contributions.

148. This includes assistance with travel fares, council tax relief, exemption from road tax, free dental care, free glasses and free prescriptions, and social services assistance.

149. This will pay for cold weather, funeral and maternity expenses, ie exceptional expenses.

150. This is paid to a person between the ages of 5 and 65 who requires care and is unable to walk for 3 months.

151. The drug of choice for neuropathic pain is:

    A amitryptiline
    B capsaicin
    C carbamazepine
    D gabapentin
    E tramadol

152. A 40-year-old woman presents with a swollen left wrist. She works as a hotel maid. On examination, there is swelling over the styloid process of the radius with pain on forced flexion and adduction of the thumb. The **single** most likely diagnosis is:

    A carpal tunnel syndrome
    B De Quervain's disease
    C Dupuytren's contracture
    D scaphoid fracture
    E trigger thumb

153. Select **two** correct statements regarding the 2003 NICE guidelines for the treatment of influenza A or B:

A Amantadine may be used for both prophylaxis and treatment of influenza in the same household.

B Zanamivir may be used for the treatment of influenza in healthy adults.

C Oseltamivir is recommended for the treatment of influenza A or B in at-risk patients who can start on treatment within 48 hours of symptom onset.

D Zanamivir is recommended for patients over the age of 60 who can start on treatment within 72 hours of symptom onset.

E Patients with diabetes are included in the at-risk patient group for influenza.

154. Select two correct statements regarding smallpox:

A In light of the threat of pox virus being used as a terrorist weapon, mass immunization is needed.

B The smallpox virus was certified by the World Health Organization as eradicated in 1979.

C In the event of an outbreak, the Department of Health plans to contain and ring-vaccinate, isolating and vaccinating contacts.

D According to the DoH, all healthcare personnel across the UK are being offered vaccination.

E Variola virus is an RNA virus.

155–159. Asylum or refugee status definitions

A asylum seeker
B exceptional leave to enter
C exceptional leave to remain
D family reunion
E refugee status
F refusal

Match the following definitions with the terms above:

155. One spouse and children of that marriage under the age of 18 are given indefinite leave to remain.

156. The Home Office accepts there are strong reasons why the person should not return to his or her country of origin.

157. A person who has submitted an application for protection under the 1951 Geneva Convention and is waiting for their claim to be settled by the Home Office.

158. A person who is granted indefinite leave to remain – permanent residence in the UK – and is eligible for family reunion.

159. A discretionary status for varying periods depending on age and other circumstances. The person is expected to return if the situation in the country of origin improves.

160. Select **two** correct statements regarding low back pain:

A Lumbar disc prolapse most commonly affects the 30- to 40-year-old age group.
B Two weeks bedrest is a first-line treatment option.
C Surgical discectomy for prolapsed lumbar disc is much more effective than chymopapain injections.
D Patients with concomitant urinary retention should be referred urgently for spinal decompression.
E Lumbar spine x-ray is often useful in the acute setting.

161. Select **two** correct statements regarding MMR vaccination:

A The MMR vaccine is not safe in children who have had an anaphylactic reaction to eggs.
B The UK recommends two doses of MMR in childhood.
C The MMR vaccine is associated with autistic enterocolitis.
D The MMR vaccine contains live, attenuated viruses.
E Children with leukaemia are at high risk and should be offered the MMR vaccine.

162. Select **two** correct statements regarding methotrexate:

A It may induce pneumonitis.
B It is usually prescribed once weekly.
C Folinic acid is used to counteract the folate-agonist action of methotrexate and is given 24 hours prior to methotrexate.
D Any profound drop in white cell or platelet count calls for immediate reduction of methotrexate dose.
E Patients require weekly full blood count and renal and liver function tests while on methotrexate.

163. Select **two** correct statements regarding Parkinson's disease:

   A Non-smokers have a 60% reduction in risk of Parkinson's disease compared with cigarette smokers.
   B Non coffee drinkers have a 30% reduction in risk compared with coffee drinkers.
   C Levodopa in combination with dopa-decarboxylase inhibitor is the treatment of choice.
   D Antimuscarinic drugs improve tardive dyskinesia.
   E Parkinson's disease is associated with a 4–6 Hz tremor, most marked at rest.

164. The following steps should be taken in the management of peripheral artery disease in primary care **except**:

   A Screen for type 2 diabetes.
   B Prescribe aspirin 75 mg daily.
   C All patients should be on a statin to achieve a 25% reduction in cholesterol.
   D Prescribe cilostazol for the first 3–6 months.
   E Consider ACE inhibitors in all patients, even if normotensive.

165. Select **two** correct statements regarding plantar fasciitis:

   A Pain may be elicited on palpation 4 cm anterior to the heel.
   B A bony spur projecting forwards from the undersurface of the calcaneal tuberosity is often seen on x-ray.
   C Steroid injections are the mainstay of treatment.
   D Stretching exercises to the Achilles tendon may be helpful.
   E Patients should be referred to orthopaedic outpatient clinic.

166. Which of the following questionnaires is used to assess postnatal depression?

   A Beck
   B CAGE
   C Edinburgh
   D Hamilton
   E SCOFF

167–173. Match the following studies with their correct descriptions:

A CAPRIE
B CARE
C CURE
D DASH
E HOT
F ISIS-2
G MRFIT
H SHEP
I UKPDS

167. This trial showed that increasing blood pressure increases the relative risk of coronary heart disease, stroke and end-stage renal disease.

168. This trial showed that a diet rich in fruit and vegetables, low-fat, and with reduced saturated and total fat can substantially reduce blood pressure.

169. This trial showed that low-dose diuretic-based treatment is effective in preventing major CVD events, cardiac and cerebral, in both NIDDM and non-diabetic older patients with ischaemic heart disease.

170. This trial showed that aspirin significantly reduced major CV events, with the greatest benefit being seen in all myocardial infarctions.

171. This trial showed that aggressive control of hypertension in diabetics led to a decrease in cardiovascular events.

172. This study showed that clopidogrel is as effective as aspirin in decreasing the risk of CV events.

173. This study showed that clopidogrel taken with aspirin for 6 months increases the anti-thrombotic effect of aspirin. However, the risk of bleeding is also increased.

174–177. Match the following terms with their correct definitions:

A absolute risk
B negative predictive value
C positive predictive value
D relative risk
E sensitivity
F specificity

174. The proportion of true positives correctly identified by the test.

175. The proportion of patients with a positive test who have been correctly identified as having the disease.

176. The ratio of disease incidence in the exposed versus the non-exposed group.

177. The proportion of true negatives correctly identified by the test.

178–181. Match the following studies with the most appropriate study design:

A case–control study
B cohort study
C cross-sectional study
D randomized controlled study

178. A comparison of case fatalities in patients with diabetes versus non-diabetics, following an acute myocardial infarction.

179. A study to determine the percentage of babies born to mothers treated with thalidomide who developed limb hypoplasia.

180. A survey of 5 GP practices' antiviral prescribing habits.

181. A study looking at the effectiveness of cognitive behavioural therapy versus antidepressants in the management of phobia.

182–184. Peripheral neuropathy

    A Charcot–Marie–Tooth disease
    B chronic symmetrical peripheral neuropathy
    C diabetic neuropathy
    D Guillain–Barré syndrome
    E multiple compression palsy
    F multiple sclerosis
    G systematic vasculitis

For each of the patients below, select from the list of options above the **single** most likely diagnosis. Each option may be used once, more than once or not at all.

182. A 30-year-old man presents with distal paresthesiae and distal or proximal weakness occurring 1–2 weeks after a GI infection. The reflexes are present initially but become absent within an hour. He soon loses the ability to walk and develops facial and bulbar weakness.

183. A 70-year-old woman with rheumatoid arthritis presents with rapid onset of multiple mononeuropathy.

184. A patient on cisplatin for metastatic seminoma presents with months of ataxia. He states that his gait is worse in the dark. No other members of his family have similar symptoms, claw toes or pes cavus. On examination, the neuropathy is confirmed as sensory and subacute.

185–192. Evidence-based advances in breast cancer

    A anastrozole (third-line aromatase inhibitor)
    B axillary dissection
    C fulvestrant (selective oestrogen receptor downregulator)
    D prophylactic mastectomy
    E prophylactic oophorectomy
    F sentinel node biopsy
    G surveillance
    H tamoxifen

For each of the numbered gaps, choose one option from the list above that best completes the sentence. Each option may be used once, more than once or not at all.

Hartmann et al reviewed over 6000 women with a family history of breast cancer who underwent (185)_____ and determined that reduction in death from breast cancer ranged from 81% to 94%. (186)_____ reduces the risk of breast cancer by approximately

50% in *BRCA1* carriers. (187)_____ has fewer complications than (188) _____ and is contraindicated in cases of pregnancy, multi-centric carcinoma and suspicious palpable axillary adenopathy. (189) _____ was until recently the standard first-line treatment for oestrogen receptor-positive metastatic cancer. Evidence-based medicine now suggests (190) _____ as first-line treatment in premenopausal women. In a North American trial of 400 post-menopausal women with metastatic disease recurring or progressing on tamoxifen, (191) _____ rather than (192) _____ was found to increase time to disease progression, increase rate of clinical benefit and lengthen duration of response.

193–197. Evidence-based management of lower urinary tract symptoms in men

A alpha-blockers
B 5α-reductase inhibitors
C antimuscarinic drugs
D *Serenoa repens*
E advice to reduce fluid intake in the evening and avoid caffeine
F referral for specialist assessment
G TURP
H prostatectomy

For each of the numbered gaps, choose one option from the list above that best completes the sentence. Each option may be used once, more than once or not at all.

Men with uncomplicated lower urinary tract symptoms arising from benign enlargement of the prostate should be offered (193) _____ initially. If troublesome symptoms persist, (194) _____ should be offered for 2–4 weeks. If men do not respond, cannot tolerate the side-effects or the prostate is estimated to be greater than 40 ml, (195) _____ should be offered. Evidence-based medicine has shown that (196) _____ improved overall self-rated urinary symptoms from baseline compared with placebo but long-term safety has not been addressed. Men with visible haematuria, dysuria, renal failure or urinary retention should be offered (197) _____.

198. Evidence-based medicine suggests that injectable adrenaline with oral antihistamine should be prescribed for any child who has had an allergic reaction that (select 3 correct answers):

A has a history of diabetes mellitus
B has a history of eczema
C occurred on exposure to only a trace amount of allergen
D occurred in a child who has asthma that requires regular inhaled corticosteroids
E was associated with mild respiratory symptoms

199. A 2-year-old girl presents with fever of 5 days, swollen hands and feet with peeling of the fingers and toes, strawberry tongue, cracked lips, non-tender cervical lymphadenopathy and a polymorphous truncal rash. Select the **two** best forms of treatment for this girl:

A aciclovir suspension
B aspirin
C Calpol
D IV benzylpenicillin
E IV immunoglobulin

200. Urgent referrals to secondary care for depression should be made in which **four** of the following cases:

A postnatal depression
B depression with hallucinations
C child sexual abuse survivors
D expressed suicidal intent
E personality disorder
F severe retarded depression
G depression in association with epilepsy
H elderly patients over the age of 65 with a first episode of depression

New MCQ Module Paper Two: Answers

1. A

2. F

3. E

4. E

5. BD

6. BCE

7. D   Both alendronic acid and risedronate (both bisphosphonates) are available as once-weekly preparations, which is more amenable for patients who dislike daily tablets. The classic Dowager's Hump is pathognomonic for severe osteoporosis without imaging. A lateral back x-ray should be obtained if osteoporosis is suspected and confirmed by DEXA scan. A value 2.5 standard deviations or more below the young adult female value is the WHO definition of osteoporosis. It is indefensible in a court of law if you do not put your patient on osteoporosis prophylaxis if you prescribe long-term corticosteroids. Recent evidence shows that repeated short courses of steroids may be more detrimental than long-term regular steroids! HRT is no longer recommended as prophylaxis against osteoporosis, and should only be prescribed for 2–3 years maximum, for relief of troublesome menopausal symptoms.

8. ABCD   Caution should be used in patients with DM.

9. ACE   Anthrax has an incubation period of 1–7 days. It is a Gram-positive rod diagnosed in cultures from skin or nasal swabs or blood cultures. Three forms of disease include cutaneous (95%), pulmonary and ingestion. Cutaneous anthrax results in a black eschar (malignant pustule) 4–9 days after exposure. Oedema, fever and hepatosplenomegaly may also be present. This form responds to oral ciprofloxacin. Only those directly exposed to spores should be given 60 days of oral ciprofloxacin 500 mg bd. CXR findings with pulmonary anthrax include widened mediastinum, lymphadenopathy and haemorrhagic mediastinitis. These findings can also occur with tuberculosis. The prognosis is poor.

10. ABCDE Other notifiable diseases include anthrax, diphtheria, dysentery, Ebola virus, encephalitis, leprosy, leptospirosis, malaria, meningitis, meningococcal sepsis, mumps, ophthalmia neonatorum, plague, poliomyelitis, rabies, relapsing fever, rubella, tetanus, tuberculosis, typhus, viral haemorrhagic fevers (including Lassa fever), whooping cough and yellow fever.

11. B Acute otitis media in a child under 2 years of age should be treated with antibiotics within 48 hours of onset of signs and symptoms of middle ear inflammation, especially with a T of 39°C or greater. Observation is recommended for children over 6 months with an uncertain diagnosis, mild otalgia and $T < 39$°C. In children aged 2 years and older, antibiotics are only indicated in severe illness (moderate to severe otalgia or high fever with a certain diagnosis of otitis media).

12. BCDE The British Heart Foundation published a fact-file sheet on CHD and air travel in December 2002. At 5,000 feet, due to the barometric pressure, PaO_2 on air is only 75 mmHg. At 8,000 feet, this figure is only 65 mmHg. The oxygen dissociation curve of normal haemoglobin allows for 90% saturation of haemoglobin at cabin altitudes, but for patients with CHD where tissue perfusion is inadequate, this poses a problem. Further information can be obtained from www.bhf.org.uk/factfiles.

13. B

14. CDE In 2000, the RCP published evidence-based guidelines for the management of stroke. Aspirin should only be started after a CT scan of the head has excluded haemorrhage. Aspirin is indicated for ischaemic stroke. Dipyridamole is offered to patients already on aspirin. Thrombolysis is not routinely offered in the UK, unlike the US. Heparin prophylaxis is also indicated for prior thromboembolism. Heparin is also offered to patients with carotid artery dissection. Blood pressure is often high after a stroke, and is only treated if it persists. About 75% survive an acute stroke and progress to rehab. Secondary prevention includes smoking cessation, reduction in alcohol and salt intake, minidose aspirin, and statins, if the patient is under 75 with evidence of carotid atheroma or h/o CHD. Patients with carotid artery stenosis or occlusion identified by carotid duplex studies may be offered endarterectomy.

15. A

16. D

17. C   The Simvastatin Survival Study was the first trial of LDL-cholesterol lowering with statins for secondary prevention of CHD.

18. E

19. B   Cholesterol and Recurrent Events (CARE).

20. ABCDE   The British Renal Association recommends referral if the serum creatinine is > 150 µmol/l. Renal function should be monitored in patients on ACEI or angiotensin receptor II inhibitors to exclude renal artery stenosis. Many patients with occult atheromatous renal artery disease may end up with renal failure requiring dialysis.

21. ABD   Sibutramine requires close monitoring of BP. Orlistat is associated with GI side-effects.

22. A

23. E

24. B

25. D

26. F

27. G

28. B

29. E

30. D

31. C

32. A   Actual ECGs are popular in the new MCQ paper. Make sure you can differentiate between these 3 conditions on ECG.

33. C

34. B

35. ABDE   To reduce pressure on echocardiography services, NICE has implemented guidelines regarding NT-proBNP blood tests for heart failure. ACE inhibitors (ie enalapril) and not angiotensin receptor blockers (ARBs) are recommended as first-line therapy for CHF. Renal function must be monitored at the start of treatment and 2–3 weeks following when initiating ACE inhibitor therapy. Loop diuretics are also recommended as first-line therapy. ValHeFT (Valsartan in Heart Failure Trial) showed that ARBs may have a role in CHF in patients who are intolerant to ACE inhibitors and beta-blockers. Beta-blockers show their effect with chronic use, and patients should be encouraged to persist with therapy. Use a lower dose in the elderly.

36. A   There is limited evidence that the cessation of cow's milk reduces baby colic, but this is a popular MRCGP question.

37. E

38. B   This woman has iron-deficiency anaemia secondary to menorrhagia from fibroids.

39. C   This woman may have ITP (idiopathic thrombocytopenic purpura).

40. B   This man may have haemochromatosis, which is often asymptomatic. Ferritin will be raised and LFTs deranged.

41. C   This boy may have Henoch–Schönlein purpura. The platelet count will be normal, since the defect is with the vasculature.

42. D   This elderly man may have multiple myeloma diagnosed by monoclonal globulin spike on serum electrophoresis, plasmacytoma on tissue biopsy or bone marrow plasmacytosis with > 30% plasma cells.

43. ABCDE NICE guidelines (October 2002) now advocate that type 2 diabetic patients also be tested annually for microalbuminuria and, if present with a BP > 140/80 then antihypertensive medication should be commenced. Statins and fibrates should be used to decrease total cholesterol and triglycerides to below 5.0 mmol/l and 3.0 mmol/l respectively.

44. C Dietary advice should always be offered with advice on lifestyle changes. It is important to assess CHD risk, since this will influence management. CHD risk factors include FHx of IHD, smoking, hypertension, diabetes, cerebrovascular or peripheral vascular disease, or severe obesity. The British Hyperlipidaemia Association advocate a total cholesterol below 5 mmol/l and TG below 2.3 mmol/l. This patient's fasting lipid results are borderline. Referral to specialist lipid clinics is advised if the total cholesterol level is > 7.8 mmol/l or the triglycerides are > 4.5 mmol/l (risk of acute pancreatitis).

45. A An FSH level > 30 IU/l with amenorrhoea is diagnostic of the menopause. HRT is now advocated for 2–3 years only, and only for relief of distressing menopausal symptoms. HRT does not offer protection against osteoporosis or heart disease as has been suggested in the past.

46. ABCDE Other risk groups for osteroporosis include patients with thoracic kyphosis, primary hypogonadism, previous fragility fracture, radiographic evidence of osteopenia, and chronic disorders associated with osteoporosis.

47. A In children under 10 years of age, only 10% with glandular fever will have a positive monospot test. Also antibodies in glandular fever are transient and peak during the first 2 weeks after clinical onset. So adults may not develop a positive monospot test until a week later. If EBV is strongly suspected in a patient with a negative monospot test, an immunofluorescence test is suggested for EBV-specific IgM or EBV serology for anti-EBNA1 IgG.

48. B Rhinolast spray is useful for children aged 2–12 who suffer from allergic rhinitis. Senile watery rhinorrhoea is a non-allergic form of rhinitis.

49. E Again this spray is for non-allergic rhinitis. Patients with nasal polyps should be commenced on a 2- or 3-month course of Betnesol drops. Larger polyps warrant a short course of corticosteroids and referral to ENT for a preop CT scan of the sinuses.

50. ABCDE   According to the British Heart Foundation, Factfile Sheet 01/2003 on pulmonary hypertension, severe symptomatic pulmonary hypertension warrants treatment in its own right. Bosentan is the newest licensed treatment for PPH. Sildenafil (Viagra) is under investigation as a potential form of treatment! There are 8 National Specialist Centres in the UK for the management of pulmonary hypertension.

51. D   SSRIs can be used as first-line therapy, although they may be slow to act. TCAs are often used for depression in the elderly, but have numerous side-effects – dry mouth, constipation, night sweats, drowsiness, dizziness, vivid dreams and fine tremor. Patients with cardiac arrhythmias on TCAs or with poorly controlled epilepsy should be offered SSRIs.

52. C   Olanzapine is an atypical antipsychotic without the extrapyramidal side-effects of the older dopamine-blocking drugs. Clozapine is reserved for treatment of refractory schizophrenia and should only be administered in hospital. Piportal depot injections are reserved for patients who are unreliable with oral therapy.

53. D   Acute pyelonephritis is associated with pyuria, >100,000 E. coli.

54. C   Transitional cell carcinoma of the bladder is associated with microscopic haematuria and a sterile pyuria.

55. E   Diabetes insipidus is associated with low urine osmolality.

56. A   Renal calculus presents with severe colic and gross haematuria. It may be associated with a UTI.

57. B   Renal tuberculosis presents with dysuria, haematuria and sterile pyuria.

58. DE   It is now recommended NOT to bathe prior to treatment. Transmission is through direct skin contact and symptoms result from an immune reaction to the mites' saliva and faeces.

59. AB   Clothing lice are not treated with insecticides. They live in clothing and will die if clothing is not worn for 3 days or more. However, they can survive in clothes worn for long periods of time. Treatment is a shower or bath and by washing infested clothing and bedding in hot water > 60°C.

60. B   The Mirena coil (levonorgestrel-releasing IUS) has an added benefit of reducing menstrual flow and dysmenorrhoea. Its contraceptive effect is by inducing endometrial atrophy and a hostile cervical mucus.

61. C   This woman may have emergency contraception in the form of Levonelle-2 up to 72 hours after UPSI. After that, the copper coil is recommended for emergency contraception for UPSI up to 5 days prior.

62. H

63. F   The COC can also be offered to patients with endometriosis (tricycling) to control symptoms.

64. D   This form of contraception is very popular in young women who can be forgetful and miss pills. Diarrhoea, vomiting and antibiotics all affect the efficacy of the pill. The POP, if offered, must be taken within the same 3-hour window each day!

65. I   This woman can be offered either LAM for the first 6 months postpartum as long as she is amenorrhoeic and is fully breastfeeding, or she can be offered Depo-Provera or POP.

66. G

67. D

68. B

69. E   COX-2 inhibitors are contraindicated in patients with heart failure. Methotrexate should be prescribed at 7.5 mg once weekly with 5 mg of folic acid weekly for potential mucosal or GI side-effects. MTX requires regular FBC, U/E and LFTs.

70. F

71. C   According to the National Disease Surveillance Centre, vomit should be cleaned with a dilute bleach solution (0.1% hypochlorite) to ensure destruction of the Norwalk-like virus (NLV), which is transmitted through the vomit of an infected individual. Sodium perborate is an antiseptic mouthwash and is similar to hydrogen peroxide and chlorhexidine.

72. ABCDE   Antiphospholipid syndrome occurs with SLE and requires close supervision during pregnancy. Mothers are commenced on aspirin and may require SC heparin or warfarin. The baby is at risk of placental insufficiency, IUGR and fetal death.

73. E   Clinical features that warrant urgent breast clinic referral include a discrete lump in a patient over 25, localized persisting nodularity in a patient over 30, bloodstained nipple discharge associated with a mass at any age, acquired skin dimpling or unilateral nipple inversion, persisting unilateral nipple ulceration or eczema, or persisting signs of sepsis in a non-lactating breast.

74. F

75. E   This woman may have primary biliary cirrhosis – a slow, chronic liver disease.

76. B   This man most likely has haemochromatosis. The definitive investigation is liver biopsy. Diabetes should be excluded in this patient.

77. A   This man most likely has a stone in the common bile duct.

78. D   This farmer may have extrinsic allergic alveolitis. Treatment is removal of allergen, oxygen, IV hydrocortisone and oral prednisolone.

79. E   This man is presenting with signs of heart failure, and would benefit from an ACE inhibitor.

80. F   This man would benefit from a trial of salbutamol.

81. D   This man may have sarcoidosis.

82. C   Tickly cough is a side-effect of ACE inhibitors, in which case angiotensin II-receptor antagonists may be substituted.

83. B   This man will most likely have an atypical pneumonia. If the infection does not clear, he may need a chest and hand x-ray to exclude tuberculosis.

84. A   Age is no bar to holding a licence. A 3-year license is issued as long as the patient at age 70 confirms with the DVLA that no medical disability is present.

85. E   Persistent BP of 180/100 or greater disqualifies a group 2 entitlement driver.

86. F   The DVLA must be notified and driving cease if cerebral metastases are present.

87. C   If the operation required was a craniotomy, the patient would be barred for 12 months.

88. A   Colour blindness is no bar to driving.

89. E   A drug misuser is automatically disqualified for a minimum of 12 months. However, with close supervision on a methadone programme, he may reapply subject to annual medical review and favourable assessment.

90. A   A single confirmed episode of transient global amnesia is no bar to group 2 entitlement. However, if 2 or more episodes occurred, driving would be banned until investigated further.

91. B   Corticosteroids induce remission in > 90% of children.

92. E   There is a poor response to corticosteroids (10–30%). Cyclophosphamide or ciclosporin may be used.

93. G   Other associations include malignancy, drugs, autoimmune conditions and infections. Treatment involves corticosteroids and chlorambucil (Ponticelli regimen).

94. I   Treatment involves high-dose corticosteroids, cyclophosphamide ± plasma exchange or renal transplant. Prognosis is poor if the initial serum creatinine level is > 600 μmol/l.

95. F   There is no treatment, and half will progress to endstage renal failure.

96. ABD   HRT is associated with increased risk of endometrial cancer after 5 years of sequential use. Raloxifene (the first SERM) is not useful for the management of menopausal symptoms and is associated with a 2- or 3-fold increase in VTE, but is used to treat osteoporosis. In a RCT in 7,705 osteoporotic women treated with raloxifene, the BMD was higher and the relative risk of vertebral fracture (0.5–0.7) was lower than in the placebo arm.

97. BCD   Cyproterone acetate is an antiandrogen used in the treatment of severe hypersexuality. Tolterodine is an antimuscarinic drug used to treat urinary frequency. Finasteride is an anti-androgen (5α-reductase inhibitor) that acts slowly on the size of the prostate and reduces risk of retention. Patients must be warned to use a condom, since it is secreted in the semen. Alpha-blockers are used in patients awaiting a TURP.

98. F   Saphena varix may also be associated with a bluish tinge to the skin.

99. D

100. A

101. E   This man may well have Pott's disease.

102. B

103. C   This woman may have SLE.

104. D

105. A   This woman may have primary biliary cirrhosis.

106. B   This man may have Wegener's granulomatosis.

107. H

108. E

109. F

110. B

111. D   Paclitaxel is a taxane and is the treatment of choice for ovarian cancer. Both paclitaxel and docetaxel are also used for the treatment of advanced or metastatic breast cancer as per NICE guidelines.

112. I   Trilostane has a minor role in postmenopausal breast cancer that has relapsed following oestrogen antagonist therapy. As it inhibits the synthesis of mineralocorticoids and glucocorticoids, concomitant corticosteroid replacement therapy is required.

113. ABCDE   Management of scars may be divided into leave alone, non-invasive and invasive methods. Invasive methods include surgical excision and resuture, resurfacing, peel, dermabrasion, reconstruction with skin grafts, laser therapy, cryotherapy, bleomycin and 5-fluorouracil injections.

114. C

115. E

116. E

117. BCDE   There are 4 types.

118. ABCDE   Drugs with narrow therapeutic range or modified-release preparations with different bioavailability should not be prescribed generically.

119. ABCDE

120. ABC   Nurses are exposed to glutaraldehyde when disinfecting endoscopes.

121. H

122. E

123. B

124. G

125. I

126. ABDE

127. ABCD

128. C   Only oral griseofulvin is licensed in the UK to be used to treat tinea capitis in children. Antifungal creams do not penetrate the hair-shaft.

129. ACE   Betadine shampoo and Cocois scalp ointment are not recommended in children under 2 and 6 respectively.

130. CD   Serotonin agonists (ie sumatriptan, naratriptan and rizatriptan) are used for the treatment of acute attacks. Ergot alkaloids should never be used prophylactically. They are also associated with many side-effects – GI upset and muscle cramps. Pizotifen is useful for the prevention of migraines.

131. I

132. C

133. B

134. K

135. J

136. D

137. G

138. F

139. H

140. A

141. E

142. C   Calcium channel blockers may be associated with gravitational oedema.

143. C   The flat may not have central heating, and if the walls are mouldy then concern arises as to whether there is a gas leak from poor gas maintenance also. Carbon monoxide poisoning indoors increases during winter, and the risk of dying is greater in the 2 million households that rely on solid fuel.

144. A

145. H

146. D

147. E

148. B

149. I

150. C

151. A   Starting dose of amitriptyline should be 10 mg nocte and increased slowly up to 75 mg if necessary. Carabamazepine and gabapentin are second-line drugs. Tramadol is used for nociceptive pain. Topical capsaicin has been used for neuropathic pain, but some patients cannot tolerate the initial increase in pain.

152. B Pain on forced flexion and adduction of the thumb is a positive Finckelstein's sign for De Quervain's tenosynovitis (stenosing tenovaginitis). The cause of the condition is unknown; however, wringing motion of the hands (eg drying out clothes) aggravates the condition. Treatment may involve steroid injection around the tendons or surgical decompression.

153. CE Both oseltamivir and zanamivir have been approved by NICE in 2003 for the treatment of adults at risk of influenza A or B who can start on treatment within 48 hours of symptom onset. Oseltamivir is recommended for children who are at risk. At-risk categories include patients over the age of 65, patients with COPD or asthma, DM, significant CV disease (excluding hypertension), or those with immunosuppression).

154. BC The DoH plans to offer vaccination to 350 key healthcare personnel across the UK (12 Smallpox Response Groups established around the UK) who would provide the first response in the event of a confirmed, suspected or threatened release of smallpox (a DNA pox virus).

155. D

156. B

157. A

158. E

159. C

160. CD Prolapsed lumbar disc is most common in the 20- to 30-year-old age group. The discs involved are L4/5 or L5/S1. 90% of patients are better within 6 weeks and 95% by 3 months. Gentle early mobilization and physiotherapy with analgesia is advocated. The Cochrane review from 2001 concluded that bedrest was not effective and may be deleterious.

161. BD

162. AB Methotrexate-induced pneumonitis is treated with corticosteroids. The Committee on Safety of Medicines has recommended a new warning label on methotrexate after numerous medication errors and overdosing. Methotrexate is usually given once weekly for the treatment of leukaemia, psoriasis and rheumatic disease. Folic acid is given once weekly after the dose of methotrexate to counteract the folate-antagonist effect of methotrexate. Blood tests are recommended before treatment commences and weekly until therapy stabilizes. Thereafter, patients should be monitored every 2–3 months. Any drastic drop in white cell or platelet count calls for immediate withdrawal of methotrexate and administration of supportive therapy.

163. CE The first two options are reversed. Nicotine and caffeine have been proven to play a protective role in the development of Parkinson's disease. Antimuscarinics are used to reduce tremor and rigidity, but can worsen tardive dyskinesia.

164. D Cilostazol is a useful adjunct in patients who have unacceptable symptoms despite 3–6 months of best medical treatment, and has been shown to increase walking distance in patients with claudication.

165. AD

166. C

167. G

168. D

169. H

170. E

171. I

172. A

173. C

174. E As sensitivity has 'si' in the word, a useful tip is to associate this with the word 'sick'. As specificity has 'fi' in the word, a useful tip is to associate this with the word 'fit'.

175. C

176. D

177. F

178. A

179. A

180. C

181. D

182. D Guillain–Barré is an example of acute symmetrical peripheral neuropathy, which can be fatal. Patients may not have absent reflexes in the first few hours of the disease. Treatment with intravenous immunoglobulin expedites recovery and reduces disability.

183. G Multiple mononeuropathy in a patient with a connective tissue disorder is most likely due to vasculitis. Treatment is with steroids ± cyclophosphamide.

184. B Cisplatin and an underlying neoplasm are both associated with chronic symmetrical peripheral neuropathy. Charcot–Marie–Tooth is autosomal dominant, so cannot be included in the differential.

185. D

186. E

187. F

188. B

189. H

190. A

191. C

192. A

193. E

194. A

195. B

196. D   Herbal therapy is available from health shops and may offer mild-to-moderate improvements in uncomplicated symptoms.

197. F

198. CDE

199. BE   This patient has features of Kawasaki's disease. Young children suspected of this disease should be referred urgently for prompt treatment to prevent coronary artery damage.

200. ABDF   All the other cases may be referred on a routine basis.

1–6. Evidence-based treatment of psoriasis

A acitretin
B betamethasone
C calcipotriol
D coal tar
E ciclosporin
F dithranol
G hydroxyurea
H methotrexate
I PUVB
J PUVA
K tazarotene

Match the following descriptions with the respective drug above:

1. Contains polycyclic aromatic hydrocarbons – known carcinogens.

2. Is useful for acute, generalized pustular psoriasis, psoriatic arthritis, psoriatic erythroderma and for psoriasis not responsive to topical therapy alone.

3. Is contraindicated in pregnancy but is the oral retinoid treatment of choice.

4. Has side-effects of hypertension and kidney damage.

5. Causes permanent staining of bedding and clothing.

6. Is a vitamin D analogue.

7–11. Diagnosis of facial rashes

A atopic dermatitis
B cellulitis
C contact dermatitis
D dermatomyositis
E discoid lupus erythematosus
F impetigo
G perioral dermatitis
H psoriasis
I rosacea
J seborrhoeic dermatitis

For each of the patients below, select from the list of options above the **single** most appropriate diagnosis. Each option may be used once, more than once or not at all.

7. A 4-year-old girl presents with a superficial erythematous rash with a golden-coloured crust around her nose, cheeks and mouth. She is systemically well.

8. A 20-year-old woman presents with a burning, itchy rash around her mouth. The eruption spares the skin around the vermilion border of her lips.

9. A 4-month-old baby boy presents with an itchy red rash over his cheeks. His mother suffers from asthma.

10. A 40-year-old woman reports facial flushing. On examination, she has erythema, papules, pustules and telangiectasia on the nose and cheeks. The facial flushing is made worse by alcohol and sun exposure.

11. A 20-year-old woman presents with several months of facial rash. It started out with polymorphic, red scaly plaques, and progresses to follicular plugging, scarring and hypopigmentation. The rash is made worse by sun exposure.

12–24. New GMS Contract

A actual
B additional
C essential
D GP
E less
F local-enhanced
G more
H national-enhanced
I opt-in
J opt-out
K out-of-hours
L PCT
M PMS
N practice
O quality
P weighted

For each of the numbered gaps, choose one word from the list above that best completes the sentence. Each option may be used once, more than once or not at all.

The new GMS contract is a (12) _____-based contract. It offers 4 types of services in the national menu. Normal services include (13) _____ and (14) _____. Supplementary services include (15) _____ and (16) _____. Rewards for (17) _____ is an (18) _____ service. Out-of-hours is an (19) _____ service. Every (20) _____ has to offer a national-enhanced service. Care for asylum seekers and the homeless are examples of (21) _____ service. Service to violent patients or to cover minor injuries are examples of (22) _____ service. Global sum calculation is based on number of (23) _____ patient list size. Therefore a practice with a clean list based in a high-inflation area will get (24) _____ money.

25–29. Evidence-based management of lower back pain

A Advise bedrest and NSAIDs.
B Arrange prompt investigation or referral within 4 weeks.
C Assess for yellow flags.
D Continue normal daily activities and prescribe NSAIDs.
E Emergency referral.
F Specialist referral if no better in 4 weeks after conservative management.

For each of the clinical cases below, select from the list above the **single** best management option. Each option may be used once, more than once or not at all.

25. A 50-year-old man presents with lumbosacral pain without sciatica.

26. A 56-year-old man presents with thoracic back pain and weight loss. On examination, he has structural deformity and widespread neurological symptoms.

27. A 30-year-old woman presents with buttock pain radiating down to her toes. SLR reproduces the pain.

28. A 60-year-old man presents with urinary incontinence, saddle anaesthesia and relenting back pain.

29. A 40-year-old man requests repeated med3 certs for low back pain.

30–36. Roles of Committees

    A CHI
    B Clinical Governance
    C GMC
    D GPC (GMSC)
    E LMC
    F NCAA
    G NICE
    H PACT

Match the following roles with the correct respective committee from the list above:

30. It is the sole negotiating body with the Department of Health, and is a standing committee of the BMA and represents all GPs in the UK.

31. It is a statutory body of locally elected GPs who meet monthly locally and annually at a national conference.

32. This analyses prescribing patterns and cost data for each practice and compares them with other practices in the area.

33. This committee overseas the quality of clinical governance and of services. It was established in April 2000 and reviews all types of organizations (ie GP practices, hospitals and PCTs) regarding their quality of services to patients.

34. This produces and disseminates clinical guidelines to promote cost-effective therapies and uniform clinical standards. It covers guidance on health technology, clinical management of specific conditions, and referral guidelines from primary to secondary care.

35. This is an initiative of the White Paper, The New NHS, and is a framework to improve patient care through high standards, personal and team development, and cost-effective, evidence-based clinical practice.

36. This authority assesses a doctor's performance rapidly to avoid years of suspension during an enquiry.

37. A tympanic membrane with chalky-white patches is best associated with:

    A cholesteatoma
    B chronic serous otitis media
    C noise-induced hearing loss
    D otosclerosis
    E tympanosclerosis

38. Select **three** correct statements listed on a patient's steroid card:

    A I am a patient on steroid treatment, which must not be stopped suddenly.
    B If you come into contact with chickenpox, see your doctor urgently.
    C For 1 year after you stop treatment, you must mention that you have taken steroids.
    D If you have taken this medicine for more than 3 weeks but less than 6, you may stop treatment suddenly.
    E If you have never had chickenpox, see your doctor for antibody testing.

39. Select the **single** best answer definition of the black triangle symbol in the BNF:

    A Denotes those preparations are considered by the Joint Formulary Committee to be less suitable for prescribing.
    B Identifies newly licensed medicines that are monitored intensively by the MCA/ CSM and requires all suspected reactions to be reported through the Yellow Card scheme.
    C Identifies preparations that are not available for NHS prescription.
    D Identifies prescription-only medicines.
    E Requires handwritten requests on FP10 prescriptions.

40. A 30-year-old woman requests a prescription for Dianette for contraception. Select the **single** correct answer regarding this prescription:

A The prescription should contain the female sign.

B The prescription must be handwritten.

C This pill comes in a 28-day pack.

D As Dianette is also used to treat acne, the patient will be charged private prices.

E Is contraindicated as a form of contraception in diabetic patients.

41–45. Drug misuse

A Refer to dual team.

B. Refer to in-patient detox centre.

C. Refer to specialist GP in drug misuse or community drug team.

D Prescribe methadone on handwritten FP10.

E Prescribe and maintain on current dose of diazepam.

F Introduce mirtazapine and wean off diazepam.

G Prescribe heroin.

H Ask patient to produce urine specimen on premises for urine toxicology to confirm presence of opiates.

For each of the patients below, select from the list of options above the **single** most appropriate management options, based on evidence. Each option may be used once, more than once or not at all.

41. A 40-year-old IVDA demands methadone since he wants to come off heroin. He states that he will steal if you do not prescribe methadone. (2 best answers)

42. A 30-year-old IVDA on methadone informs you that he has lost his prescription and has missed 3 days of methadone. He requests a repeat prescription. (2 best answers)

43. A 30-year-old man with a history of schizophrenia and heroin misuse presents for drug management.

44. A 50-year-old man requests Antabuse since he wishes to give up alcohol.

45. A 45-year-old woman requests a repeat prescription for diazepam. She has taken 2 mg diazepam nocte for the past year for anxiety and depression.

46. A court order for release of patient's medical records without a patient's written consent is called:

A Order of Determination
B Order of Disclosure
C Order of Discovery
D Order of Public Interest
E Order of Release of Medical Records

47. A 22-year-old man develops asthma 2 years after starting work in a bakery. The **two** best tests to confirm flour allergy are:

A RAST
B patch test
C skin prick test
D serum IgE
E chest x-ray

48. Extrinsic allergic alveolitis is a form of which type of hypersensitivity reaction?

A I
B II
C III
D IV
E V

49. A 50-year-old woman with rheumatoid arthritis is unable to tolerate both sulfasalazine and methotrexate. She has been on indomethacin for the past 3 years. The **single** most appropriate alternative treatment is:

A ciclosporin
B leflunomide
C misoprostol
D naproxen
E rofecoxib

50–54. Foot pain

A arthritis of the subtalar joint
B Freiberg's disease
C hallux rigidus
D Köhler's disease
E metatarsalgia
F Morton's metatarsalgia
G osteochondritis
H plantar fasciitis
I postcalcaneal bursitis
J stress fracture

For each of the patients below, select from the list of options above the **single** most appropriate diagnosis. Each option may be used once, more than once or not at all.

50. A 4-year-old boy complains of painful foot and limps. On examination, pain is felt in the mid-tarsal area. X-ray confirms dense, deformed bone.

51. A 45-year-old woman presents with pain on the underside of the heel. She reports that it is worse first thing in the morning and eases with walking. Walking upstairs makes the pain worse.

52. A 27-year-old marathon runner presents with pain in the shaft of the 2nd metatarsal. X-ray is normal.

53. A 20-year-old airline stewardess complains of pain in the 3rd and 4th toes. Pain is elicited on compression of the affected web space.

54. An 11-year-old girl presents with forefoot pain. On x-ray, the epiphysis of the 2nd metatarsal head is flattened, fragmented and granular.

55. Papillary thyroid cancer is most frequent in which **two** of the following decades:

A 20s
B 30s
C 40s
D 50s
E 60s

56. Which type of malignant thyroid cancer is the most common?

   A anaplastic
   B follicular
   C Hürthle cell
   D lymphoma
   E papillary

57. Risk factors for breast cancer include all of the following **except**:

   A breastfeeding
   B early menarche
   C first pregnancy > 30 years old
   D late menopause
   E nulliparity

58–61. ECG abnormalities

   A 1st-degree heart block
   B 2nd-degree heart block (Mobitz type I–Wenckebach phenomenon)
   C 2nd-degree heart block (Mobitz type II)
   D 3rd-degree heart block
   E left bundle branch block
   F right bundle branch block
   G Wolff–Parkinson–White syndrome

   For each of the ECG findings below, select from the list above the **single** most appropriate diagnosis:

58. The initial PR interval is normal but progressively lengthens with each successive beat until AV transmission is blocked completely and the P-wave is not followed by a QRS complex. The cycle then repeats itself.

59. The PR interval is uniformly prolonged in each cycle. All P-waves are followed by a QRS complex and the PR interval remains constant.

60. The QRS is > 0.12 s with inverted T-waves in leads I, AVL and V5–6.

61. The PR interval is constant, but not all P-waves are followed by a QRS complex.

62. The NSF for diabetes has suggested that the ideal target HbA1C should be less than:

A 5%
B 5.5%
C 6%
D 6.5%
E 7%

63–66. Oral hypoglycaemics

A α-glucosidase inhibitor
B biguanide
C glitazones
D post-prandial glucose regulators
E sulphonylureas

Match the class of oral hypoglycaemic agents with their correct primary mode of action. Each option may be used once, more than once or not at all.

63. Decreases hepatic glucose production.

64. Stimulates insulin secretion by β-cells (2 answers).

65. Delays absorption of carbohydrate.

66. Decreases insulin resistance and resensitizes the body to its own insulin

67. Which **two** statements are correct regarding treatment of vulvo-vaginal candidiasis, based on evidence?

A Treating a woman's male sexual partner significantly improves resolution of the woman's symptoms and reduces the rate of symptomatic relapse.
B Oral itraconazole has been associated with reports of heart failure.
C Oral ketaconazole requires baseline serum liver function tests.
D Oral fluconazole may be prescribed as a single dose of 150 mg.
E Nystatin pessaries should be inserted at night for at least 7 days.

68–73. Antithrombotic therapy in peripheral vascular disease

    A aspirin or clopidogrel
    B heparin and angioplasty
    C consider warfarin
    D intravenous heparin and emergency surgery intervention
    E consider aspirin plus dipyridamole
    F intra-arterial thrombolysis or early surgery

For each of the clinical conditions below, select from the list above the **single** most appropriate form of antithrombotic therapy. Each option may be used once, more than once or not at all.

68. Carotid endarterectomy.

69. Symptomatic carotid stenosis but unfit for surgery.

70. Embolic arterial occlusion.

71. Intermittent claudication.

72. Diabetes.

73. Acute or chronic arterial occlusion.

74. Which of the following is **not** a test for female infertility:

    A serum FSH taken between days 2 and 5 of the menstrual cycle
    B. serum LH taken 5–10 days before menstruation
    C. serum progesterone taken 5–10 days prior to menstruation
    D serum TSH
    E serum prolactin

75. Patients with heart failure due to left ventricular systolic dysfunction should be treated with which **three** classes of drugs (unless contraindicated)?

    A ACE inhibitor
    B angiotensin II-receptor antagonist
    C beta-blocker
    D diuretic
    E spironolactone

76. Maximum predicted heart rate is calculated as _____ minus the patient's age for men:

A 200
B 210
C 220
D 230
E 240

77. The following are components of Good Medical Practice **except**:

A In an emergency, wherever it may arise, you must offer anyone at risk the assistance you could reasonably be expected to provide.
B You should offer an apology, when appropriate, if a patient under your care has suffered harm.
C You should inform the patient, orally or in writing, why you have decided to end the professional relationship.
D You may end a relationship with a patient solely on the basis of a complaint about you.
E If you have grounds to believe that a doctor is putting patients at risk, you must inform the primary care trust.

78. According to the Royal College of Obstetrics and Gynaecology and the GMC, chaperones should be offered for which of the following cases:

A a male doctor performing a PV exam in a female patient
B a female doctor performing a PV exam in a female patient
C a female doctor performing a PR exam on a male patient
D a male doctor performing a PR exam on a male patient
E a female doctor examining a female patient's breasts

79. A 40-year-old woman presents to your evening surgery with an acute exacerbation of asthma. Her usual peak flow is 390 LPM. Her predicted peak flow is 440 LPM. Her peak flow now is 200 LPM. Her current inhalers are salbutamol and Seretide 500. The RR is 20 and pulse 96. On chest examination, there are bilateral wheezes and tightness. She has audible wheezes and is SOB at rest. The **single** most appropriate treatment is:

A Prescribe a 7-day course of 30 mg of prednisolone od.
B Start nebulizer treatment with salbutamol and ipratropium.
C Call 999 for a blue light ambulance.
D Prescribe a volumatic spacer and instruct her to put 12 puffs of salbutamol into the spacer and inhale.
E Prescribe a week's course of amoxicillin and prednisolone.

80. A 45-year-old patient with NIDDM on metformin continues to have an HbA1C of 9 for 6 months despite drug compliance. His BMI is 30. According to evidence-based medicine, the **single** most appropriate step is to:

A offer sibutramine
B add glitazone
C add acarbose
D convert to insulin therapy
E change to sulphonylurea

81. A 13-year-old girl presents with mild acne vulgaris. The single most appropriate treatment is:

A benzoyl peroxide
B Dianette
C isotretinoin
D oral doxycycline
E oxytetracycline

82. The following statements regarding acute cholecystitis are correct **except:**

A It is most often caused by gallstones.
B Percutaneous cholecystostomy is a safe alternative to cholecystectomy for those unfit for a GA.
C Patients suspected of having acute cholecystitis should be referred to hospital immediately.
D Delayed or 'interval' surgery is preferable to early cholecystectomy.
E First-line treatment includes nil by mouth, IV fluids and analgesia.

83. The following statements regarding treatment of generalized anxiety disorder are correct **except:**

A Buspirone improves symptoms in the long term.
B Cognitive therapy focuses on patients' current problems and not their past.
C There is no significant difference between paroxetine and venlafaxine in reducing symptoms in the short term.
D Benzodiazepines have been implicated in up to 10% of road traffic accidents.
E The best treatment of all is cognitive therapy.

84. Presentations for head and neck cancer include all of the following except:

A cervicalgia
B cervical lymph node enlargement
C dysphagia
D earache
E hoarseness

85–90. Headaches

A cluster
B idiopathic intracranial hypertension
C intracranial tumour
D medication overuse
E meningitis
F migraine
G primary angle closure glaucoma
H subacute carbon monoxide poisoning
I subarachnoid haemorrhage
J temporal arteritis
K tension

For each of the patients below, select from the list of options above the **single** most likely diagnosis:

85. A 45-year-old bus driver reports a tightness around his head, spreading into the neck. It lasts a few hours at a time.

86. A 20-year-old heavy smoker reports spells of headaches lasting 2–3 months each year. He has pain around his left eye, mostly at night. He has to bang his head against the wall, since the pain is intolerable. The pain lasts for an hour. On examination, the eye is red and watering with blocked nose.

87. A 55-year-old woman reports persistent headache, worse at night. On examination, there is marked scalp tenderness.

88. A 50-year-old woman reports headache, nausea and mild eye pain and sees coloured haloes around lights.

89. A 25-year-old woman reports headaches, nausea, vomiting, giddiness, dimness and double vision. She and her husband are renovating an old property.

90. A 50-year-old man complains of severe headache and neck stiffness after a stag night. It is now the worst he has ever had.

91. Which **three** of the following are cardinal signs of glaucoma?

A increased intraocular pressure
B optic disc cupping
C proptosis
D squint
E visual field constriction

92. Which **single** best treatment is advised for acute cluster headache?

A analgesia
B ergotamine
C lithium carbonate
D methysergide
E sumatriptan

93. Which **three** drugs may be used to treat menstrually related migraines?

A amitriptyline
B beta-blockers
C continuous combined oral contraceptives for 9 weeks
D mefenamic acid
E transdermal oestrogen patches twice weekly

94. The single non-invasive investigation of choice for the diagnosis of clinically suspected deep venous thrombosis is:

A compression ultrasonography
B fibrin D-dimer
C impedance plethysmography
D magnetic resonance venography
E spiral computed tomography

95. The **single** preferred imaging method to distinguish Parkinson's disease from essential tremor is:

A CT scan
B FP-CIT (DaTSCAN)
C magnetoencephalography
D MRI scan
E MR spectroscopy

96. High 'pathological' myopia is a risk factor for all of the following eye conditions **except**:

   A central retinal vein occlusion
   B glaucoma
   C macular degeneration
   D retinal detachment
   E strabismus

97. Select **two** correct statements regarding head lice:

   A Bedding must be boiled at a temperature above 60°C
   B Treatment with lotion requires two 2-hour treatments 1 week apart.
   C Infestation is heaviest behind the ears and in the occipital region
   D They are transmitted by hopping.
   E Treatment with malathion is more effective than wet-combing.

98–101. Leg swelling

   A cellulitis
   B chronic lymphoedema
   C congestive heart failure
   D deep vein thrombosis
   E ruptured Baker's cyst

   For each of the clinical cases below, select from the list of options above the **single** most likely diagnosis:

98. A 66-year-old woman complains of swelling of the entire length of the left leg. On examination, the circumference of the left leg is 4 cm greater than that of the right leg, with pitting ankle oedema. She also complains of pain and has moderate varicose veins. She has a history of atrial fibrillation and hypertension.

99. A 60-year-old obese woman presents with non-pitting oedema in both lower legs following bilateral knee replacement.

100. A 65-year-old woman presents with SOB at rest and gross dependent oedema in both legs with breakdown of overlying skin. On examination, she has an enlarged tender liver and basal crepitations.

101. A 70-year-old woman with generalized osteoarthritis presents with stiffness and swelling of the right lower leg and popliteal fossa of the knee.

102. Bulimia may be associated with all of the following **except**:

    A binge drinking
    B bipolar disorder
    C normal weight
    D score lines on the backs of the hands (Russell's sign)
    E swollen parotid glands

103. A 40-year-old woman presents with severe renal colic. The **single** most appropriate form of analgesia (unless contraindicated) is:

    A IM diclofenac
    B IM morphine sulphate and cyclizine
    C IM pethidine
    D Oramorph
    E rectal diclofenac

104. A 60-year-old woman presents with bruising. She has a history of gout. On examination, the spleen is noted to be enlarged. The white cell and platelet counts are both elevated, and there is an increase in red blood cell mass. The **single** most likely diagnosis is:

    A acute leukaemia
    B essential thrombocythaemia
    C multiple myeloma
    D polycythaemia rubra vera
    E primary myelosclerosis

105. The **single** best treatment for this woman is:

    A busulfan
    B hydroxyurea
    C melphalan
    D supportive
    E venesection

106. A 40-year-old man complains of shoulder pain. On examination, he has pain when abducting his shoulder 45° above and below the horizontal. Pain is also elicited on pushing down on his raised arm. The **single** most likely diagnosis is:

    A adhesive capsulitis
    B cervical spondylosis
    C glenohumeral subluxation
    D injury of the spinal accessory nerve
    E rotator cuff tendonitis

107. Psoriasis may be exacerbated by all of the following factors **except**:

A alcohol
B beta-blockers
C NSAIDs
D sunlight
E tonsillitis treated with antibiotics

108–112. Treatment for conditions of the nails

A Dovonex scalp application to nails
B gentamicin ear drops
C gloves and moisturizer
D Lamisil
E Sporanox
F topical steroid

For each of the conditions below, select from the list above the **single** most effective treatment:

108. Lamellar splitting.

109. *Candida* paronychia.

110. Pseudomonal nail infection.

111. Psoriasis nails.

112. Irritant hand eczema.

113–120. Treatment for dermatological conditions

A DuoDERM
B Efudix (topical 5-FU)
C Epaderm + Cocois
D intradermal triamcinolone
E iontophoresis
F Mepiform
G Mepitel
H prednisolone
I PUVA

For each of the dermatological conditions listed below, select from the options above the **single** most effective treatment:

113. Palmar hyperhydrosis.

114. Granuloma annulare.

115. Keloid.

116. Bowen's disease on the lower leg.

117. Actinic keratosis.

118. Pityriasis capitis.

119. Venous ulcer.

120. Bullous pemphigoid.

121–127. Statistics

    A absolute risk
    B attributable risk
    C mean
    D median
    E mode
    F negative predictive value
    G numbers needed to treat
    H odds ratio
    I   positive predictive value
    J   relative risk
    K sensitivity
    L specificity

Match each of the definitions below with the correct term above:

121. The most common value observed.

122. The proportion of patients with a positive test correctly identified as having the disease.

123. The proportion of true negatives correctly identified by the test.

124. Incidence of disease in the exposed population divided by the incidence of disease in the non-exposed population.

125. Incidence of disease in the exposed population minus the incidence of disease in the non-exposed population.

126. The inverse of (% treated group with the desired outcome minus % controls with the desired outcome), ie 1/ARR%.

127. If pill users are at 2 × increased risk of a DVT than non-pill users, this value is 2. It is equal to (the number of pill users with DVT multiplied by the number of non-pill users with no DVT) divided by (the number of non-pill users with DVT multiplied by the number of pill-users without DVT).

128, 129. If 40 out of 200 heroin misusers in the Subutex-treated group and 4 out of 200 give up heroin in the control group, give up heroin then:

A 5
B 6
C 10
D 18
E 36

128. The absolute risk reduction % is?

129. The NNT is?

130. Select **two** cardinal signs of retinal detachment:

A coloured haloes
B curtain falling over vision
C flashing lights
D painful loss of vision
E red eye

131. Select **two** correct statements regarding central vein occlusion:

A The fundus appears like a stormy red sea.
B It causes painful loss of vision.
C It is less common than arterial occlusion.
D There is no definitive treatment.
E Visual acuity may be reduced to finger counting.

132. Select **two** cardinal signs of diabetic retinopathy:

    A arteriovenous nipping
    B copper-wiring of arteries
    C grey, opalescent retina
    D microaneurysms
    E yellow hard exudates

133. Indications for colposcopy referral include all of the following **except**:

    A HPV testing
    B 2nd occurrence of mild dyskaryosis
    C 3 consecutive inadequate smears
    D moderate dyskaryosis
    E suspicious-looking cervix

134. The following statements regarding the Mental Health NSF are correct **except**:

    A 1 : 6 patients have mental health problems.
    B 1 : 250 patients have bipolar affective disorder or schizophrenia
    C 90% of carers who live with a person with a serious mental illness suffer from depression.
    D Performance is assessed by the National Psychiatric Morbidity Survey.
    E Standard 3 makes it mandatory to provide 24-hour Section 12-approved doctor and ASW care.

135–137. Management of mental illness

    A Continue antidepressant for 2 more weeks.
    B Increase the dose of antidepressant or consider switching to another.
    C Prescribe antipsychotic.
    D Prescribe antidepressant.
    E Refer to psychiatric outpatient clinic.
    F Urgent referral for sectioning.

    For each of the patients below, select from the list of options above the **single** most appropriate management.

135. The mother of a 20-year-old unemployed man is concerned, since her son has not left his room for 3 months. The son agrees for you to visit him at home, and during your visit you find him aloof. You determine that he does not have psychotic features.

136. You are contacted by the neighbour of a 25-year-old woman. You contact the woman, who agrees for you to visit her at home. Upon arrival, you see that there is broken window glass, used syringes, beer bottles scattered on the floor. She reports that she cannot sleep, since she hears shouting voices in her head.

137. A 35-year-old man on Prozac states that nothing has happened in 4 weeks. He asks whether he can try a different antidepressant.

138. Which **five** of the following blood tests should be arranged for a patient suspected of having Alzheimer's disease?

    A B_{12} and folate
    B bone profile
    C fasting lipids
    D FBC + ESR
    E hepatitis virology
    F HIV
    G U+E + glucose
    H LFTs
    I syphilis serology
    J TFTs

139. Drug levels are required for all of the following medications **except**:

    A carbamazepine
    B ciclosporin
    C digoxin
    D lithium
    E theophylline

140. The following statements are correct regarding severe acute respiratory syndrome (SARS) **except**:
    A 20 ml of blood in a plain glass tube should be taken.
    B Chest x-ray shows changes suggestive of pneumonia.
    C The incubation period is between 2 and 7 days.
    D Early antibiotic intervention is effective.
    E There have been documented mortalities in Hong Kong and Vietnam.

141. The **single** gold standard for detecting the hepatitis C viral RNA genome is:

    A elevated alanine aminotransferase
    B ELISA-3 blood test
    C liver biopsy
    D polymerase chain reaction (PCR)

142. The following statements regarding fitness to drive are correct except:

    A A patient may be granted a licence to drive if he has only had seizures in his sleep for the past 3 years.
    B A licence may be granted for up to 3 years if a patient has been seizure-free for 1 year.
    C A diabetic patient is required to notify the DVLA if on tablets.
    D A patient with 6/10 corrected vision is not banned from driving.
    E A HGV driver who has suffered an MI is permanently banned from driving.

143–147. PV bleed

    A inevitable abortion
    B missed abortion
    C placenta abruptio
    D placenta praevia
    E threatened abortion

For each of the patients below, select from the list above the **single** most likely diagnosis:

143. A 6/40 pregnant female presents with PV spotting. On PV exam, the os is closed.

144. A 8/40 pregnant female presents with PV bleeding. On PV exam, the os is open.

145. A 14/40 pregnant female is noted to have a uterus that is small for dates. The os is closed.

146. A 22/40 pregnant female comes for an antenatal check. No fetal heart sounds are present.

147. A 29/40 pregnant female presents with severe lower abdominal pain and PV bleed.

148–150. Methotrexate

A Continue current dose of methotrexate.
B Decrease by 2.5 mg weekly.
C Discontinue methotrexate.
D Increase by 2.5 mg weekly.

A patient has been recently started on methotrexate for rheumatoid arthritis. He has regular FBC tests. For each of the results below, select from the list above the **single** most appropriate management plan:

148. The WCC was $8 \times 10^9/l$ and platelets $220 \times 10^9/l$ in October, and 2 months later the WCC is now $3 \times 10^9/l$ and the platelets $100 \times 10^9/l$.

149. The patient complains of a cough. On examination, he is afebrile and the chest is clear. The WCC is $11 \times 10^9/l$ and the platelets are $200 \times 10^9/l$.

150. The patient reports symptoms only mildly improving on methotrexate. He is still in considerable pain. The WCC is $12 \times 10^9/l$ and the platelet count is $250 \times 10^9/l$.

151. Causes of monocular diplopia include all of the following **except**:

A astigmatism
B cataract
C dislocated lens
D pterygium
E strabismus

152. Bisphosphonates are indicated for all of the following conditions except:

A inflammatory bowel conditions requiring oral corticosteroids
B prolonged oral corticosteroid use for more than 3 months
C postmenopausal osteoporosis
D postmenopausal Muslim women
E premenopausal women with a family history of osteoporosis

153. A 14-year-old boy has persistent otitis externa. He enjoys swimming. He has been using Otomize spray. The ear swab returns as *Pseudomonas aeruginosa*. The **single** best management option is:

A Advise him to continue to use the Otomize spray.
B Advise him to wear ear plugs when swimming.
C Add amoxicillin.
D Add ciprofloxacin.
E Add trimethoprim.

154. A 20-year-old professional rugby player develops infectious mononucleosis. He wants to know if and when he will be fit to go back to contact sports. The **single** best management option is:

A Advise to wait 6 weeks.
B Advise to wait 3 months.
C Advise to return when monospot test is negative.
D Arrange for an ultrasound of the spleen to exclude splenomegaly.
E Arrange for a CT scan of the liver and spleen.

155. The following are appropriate diagnostic investigations for fever following tropical travel **except**:

A CRP
B 3 EDTA samples to haematology for thick and thin films
C malaria serology
D stool for parasites and culture with mention of countries visited
E tropical serology for schistosomiasis

156–162. Statistics

A absolute
B attributable
C case-referent
D cohort
E cross-sectional
F incidence
G odds
H prevalence
I relative

For each of the numbered gaps, choose one **single** word from the list above that best completes the sentence. Each word may be used once, more than once or not at all.

(156) _____ rate is defined as the number of new cases in a given period divided by the total person time at risk during the period.
(157) _____ ratio is good to study large populations and rare diseases.
(158) _____ study looks back from disease to exposure. It gives a comparison of (159) _____ rates. (160) _____ study looks forward from exposure to disease. Both (161) ____ risk and (162) _____ ratio can be determined with this study. However, this study is time-consuming.

163. A 10-year-old girl presents with persistent productive cough for 4 months with no relief from repeated courses of antibiotics. On chest examination, she has occasional wheezes. Which **two** investigations should be arranged?

A chest x-ray
B Ventolin challenge (4 puffs through spacer) and check lung function test
C refer to paediatric outpatient clinic
D urgent referral to chest clinic for Tb testing
E sweat test

164. Prophylactic antibiotics should be prescribed in HIV-positive patients, if the CD4 count drops below:

A 100 cells/mm^3
B 200 cells/mm^3
C 300 cells/mm^3
D 400 cells/mm^3
E 500 cells/mm^3

165–168. ECG arrhythmias

A atrial fibrillation
B atrial flutter
C atrial tachycardia
D sinus tachycardia
E ventricular tachycardia
F ventricular fibrillation
G Wolff–Parkinson–White syndrome

For each of the numbered gaps, choose one **single** option from the list above that best completes the sentence. Each word may be used once, more than once or not at all.

In (165) _____, the P-waves are absent. The atrial rate is between 350 and 600 beats/min and the ventricular rate is between 100 and 180 beats/min. In (166) _____, the atrial impulses can be conducted via the accessory pathway, causing ventricular pre-excitation and broad QRS complexes with delta waves. This accessory pathway allows for very fast ventricular rates, which puts the patient at risk of (167) _____. (168) _____ is defined as 3 or more ventricular extrasystoles in succession at a rate of more than 120 beats/min. The QRS complexes are monomorphic or polymorphic.

169. A 56-year-old obese man presents with sudden onset of severe back pain. He has no signs of sciatica or urinary incontinence. BP is 150/90. Possible diagnoses include all of the following **except:**

A acute pancreatitis
B cord compression
C renal colic
D ruptured abdominal aortic aneurysm
E simple mechanical back pain

170. According to evidence-based medicine, which of the following OTC cough medicines are recommended for acute cough in adults?

A antihistamines
B antitussives
C expectorants
D mucolytics
E none of the above

171–176. Treatment of dermatological conditions

A aciclovir
B Betnovate + Diprobase + Atarax nocte
C Capasal shampoo
D Diprosalic ointment until better + hydrocortisone cream to other areas
E Elocon
F Erythroped + Differin + Dianette (triple therapy)
G Fusidin H
H Lamisil (terbinafine) crushed tablet od for 1 month
I occlusal paint
J refer for Roaccutane

For each of the patients below, select from the list above the **single** most appropriate treatment. Each option may be used once, more than once or not at all.

171. A 2-year-old boy presents with eczema over his elbows and thighs.

172. A 3-year-old boy presents with a wart on his scalp.

173. A 2-year-old girl presents with eczema herpeticum over the face and body. (2 best answers)

174. A 6-year-old girl presents with eczema over the back of her elbows, popliteal fossa and lower back.

175. A 14-year-old girl presents with severe acne over her face, arms and back. She has tried topical therapy without success.

176. A 4-year-old Afrocaribbean boy presents with scalp ringworm, hair loss and posterior cervical lymphadenopathy.

177–183. Algorithm for treatment of breast cancer

A axillary node clearance
B axillary node sampling
C ± chemo
D chemotherapy
E DXT
F ± tamoxifen
G tamoxifen
H wide local excision
I ± Zoladex

For each of the numbered gaps, choose one management option from the list above that best completes the algorithm. Each option may be used once, more than once or not at all.

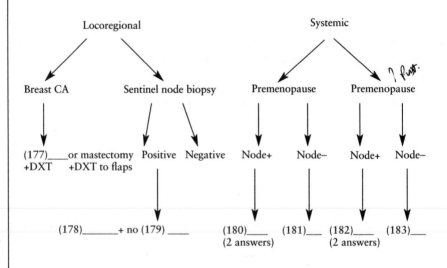

184. An 80-year-old woman requests a laxative for constipation secondary to codeine-containing analgesia. The following are suitable management options **except:**

A change analgesia to co-proxamol
B prescribe co-danthramer
C prescribe lactulose
D prescribe senna
E suggest increase fruit and bran in diet

185. The following clinical features warrant urgent referral to breast clinic **except:**

A A 22-year-old woman presents with bilateral tender lumpy breasts. She has no family history of breast cancer. She is on the combined pill.
B A 35-year-old woman presents with a persisting nodule.
C A 20-year-old woman presents with bloodstained nipple discharge associated with a 1 cm nodule. She has no family history of breast cancer.
D A 35-year-old woman has persistent right nipple eczema.
E A 30-year-old woman has a discrete 2 cm nodule.

186. The following statements regarding buprenorphine (Subutex) are correct **except:**

A It is a class C drug according to the Misuse of Drugs Act 1971.
B It should be taken at least 4 hours after last use of opioid.
C It may be used as substitution therapy for patients with moderate opioid dependence.
D It can only be prescribed by GPs with a specialist interest in drug misuse.
E Patients on methadone should be down to 30 mg of methadone od prior to conversion to Subutex.

187. The following statements regarding the NICE guidelines are correct **except:**

A GPs should not initiate therapy with acetylcholinesterase-inhibiting drugs.
B The patient should be reassessed 2–4 months after the maintenance dose has been established.
C Drug treatment may continue solely on the basis of improvement in the MMSE score.
D Patients should be reassessed every 6 months.
E MMSE score should be above 12 to consider treatment with donepezil.

188. The following are risk factors for a patient's risk of danger to others **except**:

    A past history of violence with alcohol or drugs
    B lack of remorse regarding violence
    C morbid jealousy
    D persisting denial of responsibility
    E evidence of general self-neglect

189–192. Hepatitis B serology results

    A immune, post-vaccination
    B immune, past exposure to HBV
    C infected, low risk of transmission
    D infected, high risk of transmission

    For each of the HBV serology results listed below, select from the list above the **single** most appropriate interpretation:

189. sAb +ve   sAg –ve   cAb –ve   eAg –ve   eAb –ve   DNA –ve

190. sAb –ve   sAg +ve   cAb +ve   eAg +ve   eAb –ve   DNA +ve

191. sAb –ve   sAg +ve   cAb +ve   eAg –ve   eAb +ve   DNA –ve

192. sAb +ve   sAg –ve   cAb +ve   eAg –ve   eAb +ve   DNA –ve

193. Alarm symptoms for dyspepsia include all of the following **except**:

    A Barrett's oesophagus
    B 45-year-old with positive *Helicobacter pylori* test
    C dysphagia
    D jaundice
    E PU surgery >20 years ago

194. Which is the **single** best drug of choice for social phobia?

    A diazepam
    B fluoxetine
    C moclobemide
    D paroxetine
    E phenelzine

195. The following conditions may be associated with alopecia **except**:

    A chronic iron deficiency
    B fungal scalp infection
    C hyperthyroidism
    D polycystic ovarian syndrome
    E warfarin

196–200. Contraception

    A arrange for urgent IUCD insertion
    B prescribe Levonelle-2
    C suggest Depo-Provera IM
    D suggest Mirena coil
    E switch to Brevinor
    F switch to Eugynon
    G switch to Femodette
    H switch to Micronor
    I   use condoms for a week

196. A 25-year-old woman complains of breakthrough bleeding on Microgynon 30. Her smear test, swabs and speculum exam are all normal.

197. A 17-year-old girl has had UPSI 4 days prior and seeks contraception.

198. A 35-year-old woman complains of breakthrough bleeding on Micronor. She smokes 20 cigarettes a day and has lactose intolerance. Her smear test, swabs and speculum exam are all normal.

199. A 19-year-old girl has recently had a TOP. She reports that she is too forgetful to remember to take pills every day.

200. A 40-year-old woman forgot to take her Micronor pill yesterday. She comes to you for advice. You suggest she take yesterday's and today's pills and advise that she. . .?

New MCQ Module Paper Three: Answers

1. D

2. H

3. A

4. E

5. F

6. C

7. F

8. G

9. A

10. I

11. E

12. N   The new contract is set to go live 1 April 2004, but negotiations are still in progress.

13. C or B

14. B or C

15. F or H

16. H or F

17. O

18. I

19. J Responsibility for OOHs is to be assumed by the PCO. OOHs includes 6:30 PM to 8 AM, weekends and bank holidays, and would cost GPs £6000 or 7% of the global sum calculation.

20. L

21. F

22. H

23. P This is approximately 20–25% less than actual list size and is based on a formula that incorporates age, gender, list turnover, morbidity and mortality, nursing home/residential home consults, rurality, and market forces. As of March 2003, global sum calculation based on this formula would result in many practices receiving less than in previous years – a source of great contention with the new contract.

24. E London Boroughs such as Hackney and Tower Hamlets are worse hit. Basic knowledge of the principles behind the new contract is also important for the viva. The alternative would be to remain in a PMS practice or go private.

25. D According to the RCGP guidelines reinforced by the Faculty of Occupational Medicine, bedrest is no longer advocated. The patient should resume normal activities with adequate analgesia for simple mechanical backache.

26. B This patient has a series of red flag signs (age of onset over 55, structural abnormality, weight loss and widespread neurological signs). Other red flags include non-mechanical pain, presentation under age 20, and past history of carcinoma, HIV or steroids.

27. F This patient has nerve root pain, which should resolve with conservative management.

28. E This patient has signs of a cauda equina syndrome (gait disturbance, saddle anaesthesia and sphincter disturbance) requiring urgent decompression.

29. C This man may have psychosocial yellow flags, such as a belief that the back pain is harmful or potentially severely disabling, a fear-avoidance behaviour and reduced activity levels, tendency to low mood and withdrawal from social interaction, or expectation of passive treatment(s) rather than a belief that active participation will help. Yellow flags are associated with poor outcomes. Referral for reactivation/rehabilitation should be considered in patients who fail to return to work by 6 weeks.

30. D

31. E

32. H

33. A

34. G

35. B

36. F

37. E Tympanosclerosis is an incidental finding and may be associated with past scarring of the TM. No treatment is necessary. Do not try to remove this 'cotton wool' appearance to the drum mistaking it as a foreign body, lest you perforate the eardrum! I have seen this happen in A+E.

38. ABC Also, if you have been taking this medicine for more than 3 weeks, the dose should be reduced gradually when you stop taking steroids unless your doctor says otherwise.

39. B

40. A   If you do not put the female symbol or at least write 'for COC' on the prescription, the patient will not be charged NHS prescription costs but instead private prescription charges. Without the symbol, the prescription indicates a private prescription for use for acne and not an NHS prescription for contraception.

41. CH

42. CH   If a patient has missed methadone for 3 days, he will need to be restarted on methadone at much lower doses and not his current dose, so he should not be offered a repeat prescription.

43. A   This man has a dual diagnosis – mental illness and drug misuse.

44. B   Antabuse is reserved for mantaining patients off-alcohol following an inpatient detoxification.

45. F   Some may advocate maintaining a patient on diazepam with a history of long-term use, but in the long-run slow weaning is more advisable.

46. C

47. CD

48. C

49. B   Leflunomide is a new DMD (disease-modifying drug) for the treatment of rheumatoid arthritis. It is very popular in the US and is now available on NHS prescription. Patient's BP and serum LFTs should be monitored.

50. D   Treatment is symptomatic, with foot rest or wearing a walking plaster.

51. H   Classic symptoms and treatment with steroid injection can be given in surgery.

52. J   Radionuclide bone scans will show this March fracture.

53. F Pain occurs from pressure on an interdigital neuroma, which may require excision.

54. B Osteochondritis dissecans or Freiberg's infarction presents with forefoot pain around puberty, especially in girls. Treatment involves good shoes ± metatarsal pad and limited activity for 4–6 weeks.

55. BC

56. E

57. A

58. B

59. A

60. E

61. C

62. E The NSF for diabetes was set for implementation in April 2003.

63. B

64. DE

65. A

66. C

67. BD Treatment with nystatin requires at least 14 days!

68. A

69. C or E

70. D

71. A

72. A

73. B or F

74. B   The FSH and LH tests should be performed in the early follicular phase. If > 10 IU/l, the patient should receive an early referral.

75. ACD

76. C   For women, it is 210 minus the patient's age.

77. D   It is essential that you obtain a copy of Good Medical Practice from the GMC, since MRCGP viva questions come straight from this booklet.

78. ABCDE   In July 2002, the RCOG published *Gynaecological Examinations: Guidelines for Specialist Practice*, which incorporates the guidelines of the GMC's Standards Committee and covers use of chaperones.

79. B   If her peak flow does not improve, call 999.

80. B   According to 'Treating to Target' guidance launched at the Diabetes UK Conference in 2003, a step-up treatment is advised if the HbA1C is persistently > 7.

81. A   Topical treatment is suggested for at least 3 months. Alternative topical treatment is Zineryt (erythromycin and zinc).

82. D   Vice versa is true.

83. A   Buspirone may improve symptoms in the short term.

84. A Squamous cell cancer of the head and neck constitutes 5% of all the cancers in the UK. People in their 40s and 50s are most at risk. Risk factors include alcohol, smoking and having a poor diet.

85. K

86. A

87. J

88. G

89. H

90. I

91. ABE

92. E The rest are examples of prophylactic treatment except for analgesia, which plays no role in the treatment of cluster headaches.

93. CDE

94. A

95. B

96. A

97. CE Treatment requires 12 hours or overnight treatment once weekly × 2.

98. D

99. B

100. C

101. E

102. B

103. A

104. D

105. E   Hydroxyurea is then prescribed if the platelet count or white cell count is difficult to control.

106. E   The painful arc sign is elicited between 60° and 120° of abduction.

107. D   Sunlight exposure improves psoriasis.

108. C   Lamellar splitting results from detergents, trauma or water.

109. E   Sporonex (itraconazole) is prescribed as 200 mg bd 7/7 repeated monthly for 2 pulses.

110. B

111. A   This subungual or periungual topical therapy is applied for 2 months. Elocon lotion is an alternative.

112. F

113. E

114. I

115. F   This silicone dressing is now available on NHS prescription and costs £30 for 10 dressings.

116. B Excision and grafting is an alternative treatment.

117. B Other treatment options include cryotherapy, Solease 3% (topical diclofenac), surgery or photodynamic therapy.

118. C Epiderm is a soap substitute and should be applied overnight to the scalp and washed out to descale the scalp. Then Cocois should be applied in ½ inch intervals.

119. G Mepitel is a non-adherent silicone dressing used for leg ulcers, decubitus ulcers and burns.

120. H Azathioprine may also be added.

121. E

122. I

123. L

124. J

125. B

126. G NNT, absolute risk and relative risk have all appeared in previous exams. You must know how to calculate these values given an example.

127. H

128. D 20% − 2% = 18%

129. B 1/18% = 5.56 or 6 people

130. BC It causes painless loss of vision and is an ophthalmological emergency.

131. AE

132. DE   Degrees of diabetic retinopathy increase in severity from BDR (background retinopathy distinguished by the presence of microaneurysms), pre-proliferative retinopathy (presence of lipoproteins as hard exudates, soft exudates, etc) to proliferative retinopathy with neovascularization. As new vessels are at risk of bleeding (ie vitreous haemorrhage or forming scar tissue) and may result in permanent vision loss, diabetic patients should be followed closely with annual specialist eye examinations. Laser treatment is used to achieve closure of leaky blood vessels or microaneurysms. Panretinal photocoagulation is used to treat neovascularization.

133. A

134. C   The actual value is closer to 50%. As carers are at risk of mental illness, Standard 6 is designed to cover this and suggests annual assessment of regular and substantial carers for a person on CPA. Standard 7 takes into account that 50% of suicide is due to mental health problems and ensures that staff are competent to do a suicide risk assessment. Each of the 7 standards has a designated lead authority.

135. E

136. F

137. A

138. DGHIJ

139. A

140. D   Blood should be taken during the acute and convalescent phase (14 days later) with a 20 ml sample of urine and sent to the local lab marked suspected SARS. A paramyxovirus is suspected at this stage. Cases have occurred in the UK, USA, Canada Europe and the Far East. There is no cure or prophylactic treatment. SARS is a notifiable disease of exclusion.

141. D   In October 2003, NICE will be reviewing combination treatment of once-weekly pegylated interferon. Currently the only licensed treatment of hepatitis C is interferon-α. Combination therapy involves oral ribavarin in combination with interferon-α2a or -α2b.

142. E He will be banned for 3 months as long as he is symptom-free and passes an exercise stress test.

143. E

144. A

145. B

146. B

147. C

148. C Medication errors have occurred with methotrexate. It is a once-weekly drug! Methotrexate must be stopped if any profound drop in WCC or platelets occurs.

149. A

150. D

151. E

152. E Once-weekly alendronate (Fosamax) is a convenient form of bis-phosphonate therapy. You are liable as a GP if you fail to prescribe osteoporosis prophylaxis to high-risk patients.

153. D

154. D

155. C Malaria serology is unhelpful as a diagnostic aid and is very rarely indicated. Initial investigation should always be 3 EDTA tubes for blood film. 1% of cases are now due to HIV seroconversion, which will show atypical lymphocytes on film. Suspect if patient has a rash.

156. F

157. G

158. C

159. F

160. D

161. I

162. G

163. AB   Chest x-ray should be arranged to exclude Tb.

164. B   Patients will be at risk of developing PCP, and Septrin should be prescribed.

165. A

166. G

167. F

168. E

169. B   Beware sudden onset of severe back pain in men over the age of 55. Do not forget to check the abdomen for a pulsatile AAA.

170. E   Recommendation of OTC cough medicines to patients is not justified by current evidence.

171. D

172. I   Other treatment is liquid nitrogen, which is age-dependent since it may cause some discomfort.

173. AG

174. B   If this does not work, the patient should be referred for TLO1 light cabinet for recalcitrant eczema. Diprobase should be applied while at school and Epaderm for home use. Betnovate can then be changed to Elocon when improving.

175. F   If the patient cannot tolerate erythromycin, trimethoprim may be substiuted. Triple therapy is advised for 4 months. Differin gel should be applied thinly and continued as prophylaxis.

176. H   Lamisil is prescribed according to weight. For instance, a ¼ tablet should be crushed for a child weighing < 20 kg. Treatment is od for 1 month. Apply a toothbrush briskly over the entire scalp and place in a plastic specimen cup for culture. A bacterial swab should also be taken to exclude secondary bacterial infection. To improve pick-up rates, place the swab in the culture medium first, prior to applying to the scalp.

177. H

178. A

179. E

180. DI

181. C   G3 is offered chemo, G2 is offered a chemo trial, and G1 is offered nil.

182. CG

183. F

184. C   Lactulose requires a daily fluid intake of 2 litres, or else it will cause severe abdominal cramping, and therefore should be avoided in the elderly.

185. A   This patient can be initially managed by the GP.

186. D   Any GP may prescribe buprenorphine, but it is advised that the patient also be involved with a community drug team, who will be able to offer ongoing management advice.

187. C   There has to be improvement in behaviour or function in addition to the MMSE score for continued drug therapy for Alzheimer's.

188. E   This is a risk factor for self-harm.

189. A

190. D

191. C

192. B

193. B   Guidelines for endoscopy have now changed to age 55.

194. D   Moclobemide, a reversible MAO inhibitor, should be reserved for second-line treatment.

195. C   Hypothyroidism leads to poor hair growth and a coarsening of the hair shaft. The most common cause is fungal scalp infections.

196. F   Eugynon has 100 μg more of levonorgestrel (250 μg) and the same amount of ethinyloestradiol (30 μg) as Microgynon.

197. A

198. E   Brevinor is a COC, which contains more norethisterone (500 μg) than the 350 μg in Micronor. It also contains 35 μg of ethinyloestradiol. Micronor and Brevinor are non-sugar-coated. Lactose-intolerant individuals should not be offered Microgynon or Microval, which come sugar-coated.

199. C   The IUCD is recommended for emergency contraception for up to 5 days after UPSI.

200. I

Tips on the MRCGP Written Paper Module

The written paper consists of 12 essay questions. At least 3 of the 12 questions will ask you to critically appraise a paper. The following is an outline of what you should include in your short answers (preferably in outline format with headings underlined). I have included my own set of mnemonics to remember lists, but feel free to improvize.

Critical reading protocol (mnemonic: IMROD)

I   Introduction (TBOAR)
   A   Title, author, institute (English, foreign), journal (respectable, peer-reviewed)
   B   Background (to study)
   C   Originality (idea behind the study)
   D   Aims (clearly stated). Does the study match up to the aims?
   E   Relevance (to general practice)

II   Methods (DOS)
   A   Design (longitudinal/cross-sectional, observational/experimental, qualitative/quantitative, retrospective/prospective)
     (i)   Is the study design appropriate? Repeatable?
     (ii) Are the instruments and questionnaires reliable (same result if repeated) and validated (answers the research question)?
     (iii) Are the confounding variables dealt with?
     (iv) Is there a gold standard for comparison?
   B   Outcome measures (criteria appropriate/clearly defined?)
     (i)   Are the endpoints soft or hard and appropriate?
     (ii) Are all the relevant outcomes included?
     (iii) Is it truly blind to clinicians and patients?
   C   Subjects (inclusion and exclusion criteria clear?)
     (i)   Is it representative of the population in question? Are they similar in age, sex, ethnic distribution and socioeconomic class?
     (ii)   Was there use of controls? Was the use of controls appropriate?
     (iii) Was the selection of subjects and controls without bias?
     (iv)   Is the sample size sufficient to detect significant statistical results?
     (v)   Has the power been calculated?
     (vi)   Has the sample been unchanged?
     (vii) Does the method of randomization allow reproduction of the experiment?
     (viii) Is the treatment plan clear?
     (ix)   Has the timespan been defined and is it appropriate?

III Results (TURDS)
  A Tables and graphs – understandable and clear. Is the data represented accurately?
  B Response rate reasonable (> 70%?)
  C Dropouts – have the characteristics of the dropouts (failure to respond, non-attenders) been defined? Are all the subjects accounted for?
  D Statistics – has the statistical analysis used been clear and appropriate for the design of the study? Do they include confidence limits and is the p-value < 0.05.

IV Discussion (CACA)
  A Critical evaluation of results – have the results been discussed with respect to other literature or compared with prior research? Have the applicability and limitations been discussed?
  B Aims – met?
  C Conclusions – consistent with results, justified with realistic speculations?
  D Applicability – to your population. Is it likely to change your practice?

V Others (CORE)
  A Conflicts of interest – acknowledged source of funding (pharmaceutical)?
  B Overall – clear, ethical, valid, worthwhile study. Are conclusions affordable, available and sensible for your practice?
  C References – current?
  D Ethics – local ethical committee approval?

At least 6 of the 12 written papers will ask you to discuss issues. The following is an outline of what you should include in your short answers. These buzz words will apply no matter what the subject heading!

Issues

I Issues for the doctor (mnemonic: SHIP DRS COMMUNICATIONS)
  A self-esteem
  B health assessment
  C input
  D pressure to prescribe
  E dependency
  F record keeping
  G sympathy

H   constraints of time/ chaperone
I   opportunistic health promotion
J   managing presenting problem
K   moral code
L   up-to-date practice
M   non-judgmental care/gatekeeping
N   investigations
O   consent/confidentiality
P   active listening/appraisal
Q   transcultural conflict
R   irritation of patient
S   open questioning
T   need to justify actions
U   shared care/referral

II   Issues for the patient (mnemonic: ABCD SPACESHIP)
A   awareness of danger
B   beliefs
C   chronic disease/cultural
D   denial
E   stress
F   peer pressure
G   autonomy
H   concern
I   embarassment/expectations
J   social support
K   hidden agenda
L   issues deeper
M   physical complaint

III   Issues for the practice (mnemonic: GRASP ALLOWANCES)
A   guidelines
B   review
C   audit
D   staff
E   practice formulary/partnership dynamics/practice development
plan
F   available rooms
G   local services
H   locums
I   open-access
J   written policies
K   agreed practice policy
L   nurses/nurse practitioners
M   costs of administration/changes to existing system
N   ease of availability
O   safety issues for building/handicapped access

IV   Legal and ethical issues
A   personal ethics
B   age of consent

C   informed consent
D   consult with your defence union/GMC/BMA
E   DVLA
F   Duty of confidentiality

V   Treatment issues
A   comprehensive record keeping
B   follow-up regime
C   awareness of side-effects
D   mutual agreement on therapeutic approach
E   address fears
F   implications of long-term therapy
G   lifestyle advice
H   community treatment
I   medical monitoring of drug levels
J   non-drug versus drug management
K   supportive role
L   ongoing education
M   crisis intervention
N   risks
O   share monitoring
P   Committee on the Safety of Medicines

VI Wider issues
A   local support groups
B   availability of government resources
C   cost-benefit
D   refer to colleague if need help
E   awareness of new treatments
F   making the practice adolescent-friendly
G   increased elderly coverage/demographics
H   PCT
I   Green paper to cut down on sick-time
J   NHS plan
K   new GMS contract
L   NSF guidelines/NICE
M   political – revalidation/rationing/recruitment/retention of doc-
    tors

VII Review, audit and follow-up
A   audit
B   failsafes/safety-netting
C   regular assessments
D   risk assessments
E   complaints
F   critical incidents

The written paper may have a question on screening programmes. The following is an outline using Wilson's criteria.

Screening programme requirements (mnemonic: IATROGENIC)

Important condition

Acceptable treatment for this disease

Treatment and diagnostic facilities available

Recognizable latent and early symptomatic stage

Opinions on who to treat are agreed

Guaranteed safety and reliability of test

Examination acceptable to patient

Natural history of disease is known

Inexpensive and simple test

Continuous rolling programme to be repeated at intervals

Alternatively, the written paper may ask you to come up with a protocol. The following points should be addressed in your discussion paper.

Aims clearly stated

Background – guidelines and protocols should be evidence-based

Diagnosis should be clear

Follow-up

Audit performed regularly

Responsibility for administrating or updating

Refer – when to make urgent and routine referrals; exclusion criteria

Review and update

Target group

Two of the 12 papers will ask you to cite evidence-based medicine on various clinical topics. Short of reading every weekly *BMJ* and monthly *BJGP* in the previous year, familiarize yourself with *BMJ* review articles/trials/NSF guidelines in hot topic areas. Some of the MCQs in this book have come from review articles in *BMJ*s published in 2002 and

2003! As a GP registrar, you can join the Royal College of General Practitioners as an associate member and receive monthly *BJGP*s for free. Read the contents page and make notes of any interesting hot topics. You will not be expected to cite chapter and verse, but if you can mention basic principles, and list anything and everything you have read – journals, textbooks, lectures, etc. – you will be able to fill in the empty spaces. Do not leave blank spaces.

For merit, you must quote one paper per essay question. For instance, quote the Glasgow paper that suggests giving patients 90 seconds to speak uninterrupted at the start of a consultation to say everything as a useful tool; or a 2002 *BMJ* paper that shows evidence that spending one minute of the ten-minute consultation on health promotion can make a difference. Note that it will be a different examiner marking each paper, so by all means repeat yourself.

And finally, I end my book with a copy of my approved discussion paper submission for the National Project Marking Schedule to serve as guidance as an alternative to submitting an audit project for summative assessment. It is a viable option that has been introduced recently, with scant information on guidance.

A Discussion Paper of the Issues Involved in Management of Heroin Misusers in General Practice

Summative Assessment Training Number _____

Introduction

Aims

The aim of this discussion paper is to explore the issues surrounding management of heroin misusers in general practice. This is a contentious topic, and I hope to increase GP awareness, allowing GPs to make their own decisions. Ultimately, I hope to inspire and encourage more GPs to manage heroin misusers.

Background for study

According to the Regional Drug Misuse Database,[1] the total number of drug misusers presenting for treatment with drug misuse agencies and GPs in England, during the year April 2000 to March 2001, was 118,500! The average GP may see four to eight new cases per year. The main drug of misuse was heroin. This figure is a dramatic increase from 3 years prior, when the total number was reported to be around 30,000. In 1995, the DOH instructed health authorities to establish protocols for the shared care of drug misusers. According to an article published by Gerada and Tighe in the *British Journal of General Practice* in 1999, about one-fifth of the 120 health authorities responded with differing protocols in place![2] Now there is hot debate over the new GP contract. In the 17 October issue of *Doctor* magazine, the GPC Joint-Deputy Chairman, Dr Hamish Meldrum, is quoted as stating that 'all treatment of drug misuse would most likely be a nationally enhanced service'. However, Dr Clare Gerada, Director of the RCGP's Drug Misuse Unit and a Government adviser, is urging that management of drug misuse should fall under the category of core and additional services.[3]

The problem with Dr Meldrum's comments is that there are only 400 GPs from England and 50 from Wales who have successfully completed the 5-day RCGP Certificate Level training programme in drug misuse. Placing drugs in national or local enhanced categories would put added pressures on these specialist GPs and the PCTs. Services provided by GPwSIs in drug addiction should be acknowledged with compensation in the new contract. According to Dr Gerada, 'currently, 25% of all GPs in England provide substitute medication'. With the numbers of drug misusers on the rise, the debate continues as to what role the GP should adopt with the management of drug misusers.

Hypothesis and objective

As a CLAS (Consultancy Liaison Addiction Service) SHO in a busy GP practice, I identified 20 heroin misusers. Under the guidance of a GPwSI in drug addiction, I managed these drug misusers for a period of 6 months and developed insight into the issues surrounding management of drug misusers in general practice. As a GP registrar, I have come across resistance by GPs to managing these patients in their respective practices, but I also understand the need to give fair and non-judgmental care to this neglected and growing patient population. My objective is to explore these issues, allay concerns and perhaps encourage GPs to provide minimum core services to these patients, if reluctance still persists with prescribing substitute medication.

Methods

Design

The design of this paper is to discuss the issues surrounding management of heroin misuse in general practice. Sources include discussions with GPwSIs in drug addiction, discussions with GPs reluctant to prescribe, first-hand experience acquired as a CLAS SHO, the 'Orange Book' (1999 DOH guidelines for clinical management of drug addiction)[3] and review of the current literature (*Doctor* magazine, Internet, and Medline). Articles identified by the latter used searches of the 1999–2002 databases and The Cochrane Library. Keywords used in the search were: 'heroin', 'drug addiction', 'management', 'statistics' and 'treatment'. Papers were selected based on relevance both to heroin addiction and to general practice. The papers were then narrowed down to those published in a peer-reviewed journal or by authors affiliated with renowned university institutions. Abstracts and papers were read by the author.

Subjects

Exclusion criteria for GP management of heroin misusers as identified by the Orange Book are patients with dual diagnoses (mental health diagnosis and drug/alcohol addiction), pregnancy and adolescent drug misuse. The needs of these patients should be addressed by specialist services.

Inclusion criteria for GP management of heroin misusers are registered patients who were highly motivated to cooperate with either drug maintenance or heroin detoxification therapy in liaison with specialist services (shared care arrangements with a local drug addiction team or a GPwSI).

Outcome measures

Successful outcomes in the management of heroin misusers in general practice were defined in the literature as no deaths, no drug overdoses and improvement in occupational status.[4] Short-term successful outcome in the GP setting is compliance.

Relevant findings and discussion

The management of heroin misuse in general practice can be subdivided into five issues. The first issue surrounds the doctor. As the average GP will only see four to eight new patients per year, GPs should not feel overburdened. The GP should provide core medical services to a heroin misuser. GPs express concerns over their lack of expertise. A good source is the Orange Book,[3] which offers guidelines that are presented clearly and succinctly. The history should include questions on the age of starting drug misuse, type of drug(s) misused, routes of administration, degree of dependence (quantity smoked or injected per day), habits of sharing needles or filters, identification of complications of drug misuse (abscess, thrombosis, chest infection), hepatitis B/C or HIV status with education on modes of transmission, psychiatric history, forensic history, social history, and previous attempts at rehabilitation (reason and length before relapse). These questions are straightforward.

The guidelines on examination are listed as assessment of signs of opiate withdrawal or intoxication, needle track marks, skin abscesses or cellulitis, dental caries, deep venous thrombosis, chest infections and signs of endocarditis, and mental health (risk of self-harm, depression, confusional states). Again, this checklist can be performed in a general practice setting.

The Orange Book suggests that investigations should ideally include blood for haemoglobin, creatinine, liver function tests, hepatitis B, hepatitis C antibody and HIV antibody. As heroin misusers have poor veins, GPs will be burdened with taking blood from these patients. In the initial consultation, a urine sample is requested for confirmation of opiate dependence, ie toxicology screen. The client is then instructed to return a week later for the urine results and commencement of treatment. Heroin is detectable in urine for up to 48 hours as the metabolite morphine. Again, these steps can be applied to a GP setting. The GP should also be aware of local services available for the heroin misuser – community drug projects, local drug addiction teams, specialist liver units, etc. – if he chooses not to offer prescribing services. Alternatively, if a GP is interested in acquiring further specialist training, the RCGP offers Certification in Drug Addiction.

A shortcoming with the Orange Book is that it readily admits that 'there is no single ideal model of shared care and that it depends on the willingness and flexibility of specialist services, GP and the Primary Health Care Team'. Merrill and Ruben, in 'Treating drug dependence in primary care: worthy ambition but flawed policy?' criticize these 'unclear definitions about shared care'.[5] Future developments should be made in this area; however, PCTs vary across the board and uniformity in care is difficult to achieve.

The GP may have concerns regarding his safety. According to a recent article published in the 31 October issue of *Doctor*, policies regarding protecting GPs from violent patients vary enormously across the UK from rapid-response agreements with the police in Scotland to Surrey and Sussex trusts negotiating with security guard companies. The deadline for English PCTs and Welsh LHGs to have plans in place for protecting GPs from violent patients is imminent, and hopefully this will abate GP concerns. Measures can be taken to decrease risk of violence from a patient, which include positioning in the room with a clear exit, alarm buttons under desks, and learning strategies to 'talk down' a patient both by non-confrontational verbal and body language, ie sitting sideways to the patient. As a CLAS SHO, I had two potentially violent encounters with heroin misusers. They both stood up and raised their voices in a threatening manner, but I was able to calm both patients by active listening, by acknowledging their concerns and by offering options.

The second issue involves the patient. The heroin misuser may have difficulty in establishing rapport with a GP. The misuser is afraid of the stigma of being labelled. The misuser may have hidden concerns regarding hepatitis or HIV status. Most users are not in control of their disease and have difficulty seeking help. When they do, they may face discrimination from both the GP and society. Some practices even ban heroin misusers. Casualty then takes the brunt of ad hoc visitations by drug misusers presenting with complications – deep venous thrombosis, cellulitis, etc. In my experience as a CLAS SHO, heroin misusers are normal people, housewives with children, professionals (lawyer, graphic designer, etc.), students, builders, etc. who seek help.

A third major area of concern is the issues for the practice. The practice must have an agreed practice policy. Drug misusers are unlikely to keep appointments, so flexibility is important. Designated drop-in times should be offered. The reception staff may be afraid of harassment and may even threaten to leave! Drug misusers are known to vandalize property. In one practice, the waiting room was trashed. In another, needles were left in the loo. In another, the GP's mobile was stolen from his consulting room. Patients and families may be intimidated by the presence of heroin misusers in the waiting room. GPs may be concerned that the reputation of their surgeries is compromised. Perhaps a solution is that a GP only choose to manage a small number of heroin misusers, agree to see them at designated times (beginning of a list), and adopt a zero-tolerance stance when it comes to vandalism. The patient is warned and then struck-off the list. The practice will need to be reimbursed by the PCT for offering services to heroin misusers. However, the new GP contract does not categorize drug addiction under an additional service category. This may dissuade practices from offering these services.

The fourth issue revolves around treatment. GPs may be hesitant about prescribing substitute medication. In fact, Merrill and Ruben point out that there are so few papers on evidence-based management of heroin addiction in general practice![5] Since its development in 1964, the mainstay of treatment for heroin addiction has been methadone maintenance treatment (MMT). A concern of GPs is the risk of death from topping up on methadone treatment. The most recent British papers on MMT were presented in 2002 by Keen *et al.*[6,7] A study of deaths from drugs of abuse in Sheffield from 1997 to 1999 showed no evidence that the availability of methadone is a factor in the increase in the number of drug of abuse-related deaths.[6] Keen *et al.* looked at all drug-related deaths obtained from the City of Sheffield Coroner between 1997 and 2000. Deaths attributable wholly or partially to methadone poisoning fell from 37% in 1997 to 18% in 1999 against a background of increased methadone prescribing. The subsequent study by Keen *et al.* of methadone maintenance treatment provided in a primary care setting in Sheffield to 400 untreated patients also showed no increase in methadone-related mortality: the Sheffield experience 1997–2000.[7]

An alternative mode of treatment for heroin addiction is buprenorphine, which is now being offered with successful outcomes.[4] France was the first country to promote the extensive used of buprenorphine through the primary care setting. Over 60,000 drug misusers in France have been treated with buprenorphine (Subutex).[8] Vignau *et al.* discuss the success of practice-based buprenorphine maintenance treatment (BMT) in France for opiate-addicted patients.[4] They looked at 142 patient records between 12 February 1996 (the official release date) and 31 January 1998 and followed the first 61 weeks of BMT. The treatment outcomes were no deaths, three drug overdoses and improvement in occupational status. Their conclusion was that practice-based BMT appears to be a safe and acceptable response to moderate heroin addiction. However, this paper did discover that there was a lack of physicians' training and an absence of objective measurement of illicit drug use. Nowadays, buprenorphine can be detected in the urine toxicology screen, making compliance checks possible. Buprenorphine is recommended and recognized for moderate opiate misuse by the DOH. MMT should be at 30 mg/day or less prior to conversion to buprenorphine. The only reservation I have here is the issue of cost. According to the BNF, methadone costs £3.50 for a week's course of 30 ml od. A week's course of buprenorphine (Subutex) costs £20 based on seven 8 mg tablets!

Alternative specialist treatments to MMT and BMT include naltrexone and diamorphine. Naltrexone is an opioid antagonist used in the treatment of heroin dependence. Naltrexone has been used by general practitioners in Australia for the past 2 years. Tedeschi presented a paper outlining GP guidelines for use of naltrexone (Revia).[9] My criticism of this paper would be that as this drug requires close monitoring of liver function tests, initiation should only be made by a specialist. However, naltrexone is mentioned in the Orange Book as an acceptable method of blockade of opiates. Naltrexone implants are available in the UK, but costs for 6 months of treatment can reach £5000 in the private sector.

Medical prescription of heroin has been studied in Switzerland since 1994. Brehmer and Iten from the University of Zurich presented a review paper on a group of heroin addicts who had failed all previous medical therapies.[10] They were prescribed heroin and supported by health and social services. At the end of 12 months, 76% were still compliant. This is a controversial topic, as are shooting galleries, and GPs will be resistant to this form of management of heroin addiction.

A GP also has a role in educating the drug misuser on harm minimization. Up to 90% of intravenous heroin addicts carry the hepatitis C virus

(HCV). HCV can also be contracted vertically, through blood transfusions, through acupuncture, through body tattooing and through unprotected sexual intercourse. If HCV is detected in the active, early stage (in which liver enzymes ALT and AST are elevated), the client is likely to respond to antiviral therapy.[11] HCV-positive clients should be offered hepatitis A and B vaccinations to avoid co-infection and should be advised to abstain from alcohol.[12] Non-injecting heroin users are also at risk for HCV, HIV and HBV through sexual intercourse and should be offered hepatitis B vaccination.[13] Patients should be informed of local needle exchange programmes by the GP.

The fifth issue surrounds the role of other professions. An arrangement should be made with the local pharmacist to dispense substitute medication. Issues arise for the pharmacist. Does he feel safe having drug misusers waiting around his pharmacy? How will this affect his regular customers? What are the chances of his pharmacy being vandalized, as he will be stocking methadone?

Guidelines should be established regarding the role of shared care with community drug teams or GPwSIs. At the moment, there are only 400 GPwSIs in drug addiction – too few to cover over 118,500 drug misusers in the UK. Who will fund community drug teams on a local and national basis, if the new GP contract comes to pass? Are there enough resources to cover this growing population group?

Conclusion

With heroin misuse on the rise, GPs and PCTs need to manage these patients appropriately. Drug misusers are regular people who should have their basic medical needs met. GPs who are reluctant to prescribe substitute medication should provide core medical services, offer harm-limitation advice, blood testing and information on local services, and maintain a zero-tolerance attitude to vandalism or inappropriate behaviour. Each practice must also consider the implications to the practice, staff and patients. I have presented the relevant literature on the management of heroin misusers in general practice to allay concerns GPs may have regarding prescribing. The most popular drugs for drug maintenance or heroin detoxification in general practice are methadone and buprenoprhine. Keen *et al.* have demonstrated that methadone prescribing is not associated with an increase in methadone-related mortality. Prescribing methadone as a daily-pick-up drug may also reduce overdose. GPs are being introduced to buprenorphine. Even with prescribing pressures now assumed by the PCT, the difference in cost (£16.50/week) may make GPs hesitant to prescribe this costly and yet successful alternative to methadone in moderate heroin addiction. Buprenorphine blocks the effects of heroin and therefore cannot contribute to an overdose as can methadone.

Another conclusion to be drawn from the literature is that practitioners need education. Both Merrill and Ruben and Vignau *et al.* point out that there is a lack of physicians' training. GPs who feel they lack training and would like to manage heroin misusers can obtain specialist certification, or work alongside a GPwSI in the practice or with community drug teams. But with only 400 GpwSIs, there are clearly not enough to manage all heroin misusers in the UK.

It is also evident that there is no clear shared protocol among GPs, PCTs and specialist services on how to manage heroin addiction in primary care. Even the Orange Book attests to this and explains that different areas will have different needs and resources. Merrill and Ruben flag this area of concern in their paper. Care is not uniform!

Issues also arise for other professions – the local pharmacist, community, overburdened local drug teams. A GP's decision to prescribe affects both the local community and, on a national level, relieves the burden of specialist resources.

For GPs who are still hesitant to offer even core services to heroin misusers, I suggest they visit my GP surgery, which offers substitute medication to heroin misusers with the help of an in-house GPwSI. My practice can serve as a beacon practice for visiting GPs to allay concerns. The CLAS team has also been visiting local GP surgeries to educate GPs. Writing this paper has made me aware of the many issues involved in the management of heroin misusers and its wider implications.

References to the literature relevant to the project

1. Regional Drug Misuse Database. *Statistics from the Regional Drug Misuse Database on Drug Misusers in Treatment in England 2000/01*. London: DOH, 2001.
2. Gerada C, Tighe J. A review of shared care protocols for the treatment of problem drug use in England, Scotland, and Wales. *Br J Gen Pract* 1999; **49**: 125–126.
3. Department of Health. *Drug Misuse and Dependence – Guidelines on Clinical Management*. London: The Stationary Office, 1999.
4. Vignau J, Duhamel A, Catteau J, Legal G *et al*. Practice-based buprenorphine maintenance treatment (BMT): How do French healthcare providers manage the piate-addicted patients? *J Subst Abuse Treat* 2001; **21**: 135–144.
5. Merrill J, Ruben S. Treating drug dependence in primary care: worthy ambition but flawed policy? *Drugs: Education, Prevention & Policy* 2000; **92**: 567–575.
6. Oliver P, Keen J, Mathers N. Deaths from drugs of abuse in Sheffield 1997–1999: What are the implications for GPs prescribing to heroin addicts? *Fam Pract* 2002; **19**: 93–94.
7. Keen J, Oliver P, Mathers N. Methadone maintenance treatment can be provided in a primary care setting without increasing methadone-related mortality: the Sheffield experience 1997–2000. *Br J Gen Pract* 2002; **52**: 387–389.
8. Schering-Plough Medical Information. *Subutex Dosage Guidelines*. Welwyn Garden City: Schering-Plough, 1998.
9. Tedeschi M. Naltrexone for opioid dependence. An additional tool for general practitioners. *Aust Fam Physician* 2002; **31**: 18–20.

10. Brehmer C, Iten PX. Medical prescription of heroin to chronic heroin addicts in Switzerland – a review. *Forensic Sci Int* 2001; **121:** 23–26.

11. Tennant F. Hepatitis C, B, D, and A: contrasting features and liver function abnormalities in heroin addicts. *J Addict Dis* 2001; **20:** 9–17.

12. Robaeys G, Mathei C, Buntinx F, Vanranst M. Management of hepatitis C virus infections in intravenous drug users. *Acta Gastroenterol Belg* 2002; **65:** 99–100.

13. Gyarmathy VA, Neaigus A, Miller M, Friedman SR *et al*. Risk correlates of prevalent HIV, hepatitis B virus, and hepatitis C infections among noninjecting heroin users. *J Acquir Immune Defic Syndr* 2002; **30:** 448–456.